Vision Therapy: Exercise Your Eyes and Improve Your Eyesight

Dean Liguori

Table of Contents

Preface

In 2000 A.D., I experienced physical eye trauma to one eye resulting in an injury that was compounded by an erroneous medical prescription designed to treat the injury. The combined trauma and damage caused by the prescription drug resulted in severely limited vision in my injured eye.

Unable to accept the result of this injury, I embarked on a mission to overcome it. As a result of the damage I sustained, I had the opportunity to interact with accomplished doctors in many prestigious universities and institutions. I participated in events and seminars that only doctors were invited to and engaged in all available rehabilitation. I researched and sought all information, studies, and associated work on vision impairment and restoration that I could get my hands on.

One important observation of this journey was the adherence of most of the vision industry to the medical model of healing. This failed model takes a general approach to correcting vision problems by mitigating symptoms without offering any solution to the underlying disorder.

One important discovery of this journey was the field of sequencing neurosensory and neuromuscular activities that are individually prescribed to develop, rehabilitate, and enhance visual skills and information processing. This field is also referred to as vision therapy.

My journey resulted in the restoration of my vision. The restoration of the vision of others that I shared these concepts with motivated me to develop my "Vision Therapy System" that I now share with you in this book.

Dean Liguori

Author Vision Therapy: Exercise Your Eyes and Improve Your Eyesight

ImproveYourVision.org Communications

Thank you for taking the time to read my book.

If you like what you read and are interested in more information on how to improve your vision, please go to my website and sign up for my email list.

You will be the first to know about new articles; you will receive additional vision therapy techniques and exercises, special offers, and alerts of any new editions and releases of this book.

Here is the link to my website where you can subscribe to my email list:

www.ImproveYourVision.org

I also post information and articles to my Facebook page located at:

https://www.facebook.com/ImproveYourVision

If you enjoyed my book please consider giving me a positive review if available at your selected point of purchase.

Dean Liguori

Author Vision Therapy: Exercise Your Eyes and Improve Your Eyesight

Chapter 1 Introduction

The concept of vision therapy to naturally improve your eyesight may not be as absurd as you think.

The possibility and option of improving visual acuity simply by strengthening eye focusing muscles, maintaining lens flexibility, and relieving accumulated eye stress is important for those with poor or deteriorating vision to know.

Vision therapy is a viable alternative for those who currently rely on or feel they may need corrective visual devices or surgery to read or see clearly.

For those who read for long periods of time or look at computer screens all day, this program and the exercises contained in it, are crucial to maintaining your normal vision into old age.

In hearing the term "vision therapy", or upon hearing claims that you can improve your vision using vision therapy, many questions may come to mind:

- What is vision therapy?
- Who will benefit from vision therapy?
- Do vision therapy programs really work to naturally improve eyesight?
- How is vision therapy currently being used today?
- What is the difference between an optometrist and ophthalmologist?

- Why have I not heard about the effectiveness of vision therapy?

These questions are addressed in the "About Vision Therapy" Chapter 2.

In order to understand how vision therapy can improve your vision, you must understand how your eyesight works.

In the "About Eyesight" Chapter 3, the following topics and questions are examined:

- How does your eyesight work?
- Factors that affect visual acuity
- Why does our eyesight worsen as we age?
- Common eye diseases

Chapter 4 "About Vision Therapy Programs" contains information on the following subjects:

- Three ways eyesight can be improved
- Improving visual acuity and correcting visual practices
- How corrective lenses harm eyesight
- What makes an effective vision therapy program?
- What is computer vision syndrome?
- Pinhole glasses

Chapter 5 "Additional Factors to Consider" covers additional factors to consider for an effective vision therapy program to naturally improve eyesight.

- Protecting your eyesight
- Disease

- Medication
- Aging
- Diet and nutrition
- Additional diet and nutrition resources for overall health
- Physical exercise
- Stress relief through meditation and relaxation

The final section contains my Vision Therapy System that you will use to create your own personalized vision therapy program designed specifically for your needs.

Chapter 2 About Vision Therapy

Question: What is "vision therapy"?

The American Optometric Association defines vision therapy as a sequence of neurosensory and neuromuscular activities individually prescribed and monitored by a doctor to develop, rehabilitate and enhance visual skills and processing.[1]

The definition of vision therapy includes eye exercises to develop or improve visual skills and abilities; improve visual comfort, ease, and efficiency; and change visual processing or interpretation of visual information. Eye exercises that incorporate lenses, training glasses, prisms, filters, patches, electronic targets, or balance boards may be used. The eye exercises are combined into a vision therapy program.

A physician administered vision therapy program is usually based on the results of an eye examination or consultation, and takes into consideration the needs of the patient and the patient's signs and symptoms. It can also take into consideration the results of any standardized tests that are administered.

A vision therapy program prescribed by a doctor usually consists of supervised in-office and at home exercises performed over weeks to months. The length of the therapy program varies depending on the severity of the diagnosed conditions, typically ranging from several weeks or months but can be even longer periods of time.

Any non-surgical methods or activities of improving eyesight, such as eye exercise, coordination activities, use of training glasses, patch therapy, etc. is referred to as vision therapy.

Although vision therapy may not be a term that is recognized by all optometrists; orthoptists, optometrists, and ophthalmologists, all are able to use vision therapy for the benefit of their patients.

Question: Who will benefit from vision therapy?

Benefits from vision therapy can be seen by those with:

- **Age related visual deterioration**: those who are experiencing reduced quality in eyesight as a result of aging, including loss of elasticity of the lens in the eye and weakness of the ciliary muscles in changing the shape of the lens to focus and fine tune visual acuity.

- **Eyestrain**: Eyestrain is often circular or self perpetuating, and can result from poor visual practices. Those who study, read, or look at computer screens for long periods of time can create stress in the eye that can decrease visual acuity. Increasing numbers of people spend substantial amounts of time in front of a computer screen, cell phone, or other electronic devices held at close distances. Because of these practices, there are increasing percentages of people that experience eye strain, vision related headaches, the inability to concentrate, and other visual related problems.

- **Learning problems related to vision problems**: Poor visual acuity, focusing, eye teaming and tracking, and visualization skills all affect one's ability to concentrate and learn. Reading speed and comprehension, focus, and concentration can all be improved with vision therapy.

- **Performance in sports**: athletes use vision therapy to improve visual reaction time, hand eye coordination, peripheral awareness, achieve faster accommodation and increased ability to track moving objects.

- **Neurological disorders or trauma to the nervous system**: those with vision problems related to strokes or traumatic brain injuries, cerebral palsy, multiple sclerosis, developmental delays, and some types of other neurological ailments can improve their visual system.

As approved by the American Optometric Association Board of Trustees, April 2009, research has demonstrated that vision therapy can be an effective treatment option for the following:[1, 2]

- Ocular motility dysfunctions (eye movement disorders)
- Non-strabismic binocular disorders (inefficient eye teaming)
- Strabismus (crossed eye or misalignment of the eyes)
- Amblyopia (poorly developed vision)
- Accommodative disorders (focusing problems)
- Visual information processing disorders, including visual-motor integration and integration with other sensory modalities
- Visual sequelae of acquired brain injury

What outcomes can be expected from vision therapy?

When both of the eyes move, align, and fixate with the lens of each eye focusing sharply together, visual acuity improves and vision is completely redefined. Those who engage in vision therapy usually find that:

- The ability to see near or far objects improves
- The ability to track and follow moving objects improves

- Creating and visualizing mental images becomes easier
- Reading level and speed increases
- Learning becomes easier
- Concentration improves
- Athletic performance improves

For all vision problems that can be completely corrected with eye glasses or contact lenses, the sole cause of the vision problem is the inability of the lens to focus light rays at the proper location on the retina. Vision therapy can help to fix these problems. Although the rate of improvement of those engaging in vision therapy may vary, progress is usually seen very early in the vision therapy program by all, usually in the very first therapy session.

Question: Do vision therapy programs really work to naturally improve eyesight?

The short answer is YES!

Professional athletes, Air Force fighter pilots, and most recently, patients of hundreds of medical eye doctors who claim to be "Board Certified in Vision Therapy," are examples of the many people who have naturally improved their eyesight and restored lost vision by changing their visual practices and routinely performing short and simple vision therapy eye exercises.

The longer answer follows.

Vision therapy has been used since the early 19th Century. Ophthalmologist William H. Bates M. D., invented the "Bates Method", a system to naturally improve eyesight and correct blurred vision, in the early part of the 19th century. From his observations of patients with vision related eyesight problems Dr. Bates came to a number of conclusions, including the following:

- The quality of your eyesight can change, either for the better or for the worse
- Poor eyesight is caused by the strain to see
- The way to achieve better eyesight is through relaxation of both mind and body

Dr. Bates had a number of proponents as well as critics, and his methods are still debated and practiced to this day. Many optometrists and ophthalmologists have greatly expanded his treatment mythology and much more has been learned since his work was made public. There are a number of websites that provide information about Dr. Bates and the Bates Method of vision improvement. The Bates Association for Vision Education website can be found at www.seeing.org.

Dr. Bates original book "The Cure of Imperfect Eyesight by Treatment without Glasses" published in 1920, can be purchased inexpensively online or found and downloaded by using any internet search engine using the keywords "The Cure of Imperfect Eyesight by Treatment without Glasses pdf."

Question: How is vision therapy currently being used today?

Many medical organizations currently testify to the effectiveness of vision therapy and advocate the use of it. The following organizations utilize vision therapy.

American Association for Pediatric Ophthalmology

The American Association for Pediatric Ophthalmology indicates that vision therapy can be beneficial in the treatment of symptomatic convergence insufficiency.[3] Even though the age of their patients range from 0 to 20 years does not mean that the success they have with vision therapy cannot be extrapolated to age ranges beyond 20 years.

American Optometric Association

As previously cited, the American Optometric Association states that research has demonstrated that vision therapy can be an effective treatment option for the previously listed disorders.

College of Optometrists in Vision Development (COVD)

Doctors are able to achieve Board Certification in Vision Therapy.

Perform an internet search for "Board Certified in Vision Therapy" to see just how prevalent these doctors are.

Are the results of these searches just examples of doctors using effective marketing to increase business revenue by attracting patients with specific needs, or could there really be a medical "board certified" vision therapy program that can improve and restore lost vision and maintain good vision?

"Board Certifications in Vision Therapy" are provided by the College of Optometrists in Vision Development or "COVD". The mission of COVD is to serve as an advocate for comprehensive vision care emphasizing a developmental and behavioral approach. COVD certifies professional competency in vision therapy, serves as an informational and educational resource, and advances research and clinical care in vision development and therapy.[4]

To be designated as Board Certified in Vision Therapy from COVD an optometrist must complete the fellowship certification and receive board approval from the COVD International Examination and Certification Board (IECB). The fellowship process consists of; guided study, written examination, oral interview, repeating examinations, fellowship Induction, case study submissions, certified examinations, and further oral examination and interview.

Both optometrists and ophthalmologists validate and provide credibility to vision therapy by currently using it to improve eyesight

To learn more about vision therapy or the Board Certification process you can visit the link under Reference Number 4 in the References section, or use any internet search engine to search for:

- International Examination and Certification Board (IECB)
- College of Optometrists in Vision Development www.covd.org
- COVD Fellowship Certification Guide

Question: What is the difference between an optometrist and ophthalmologist?

An optometrist is a health care professional who is licensed to provide primary eye care services.

Examples of treatments are:

- Examine and diagnose eye diseases such as glaucoma, cataracts, and retinal diseases and, in certain states in the U.S., how to treat them
- Diagnose related systemic conditions such as hypertension and diabetes that may affect the eyes
- Examine, diagnose and treat visual conditions such as nearsightedness, farsightedness, astigmatism and presbyopia
- Prescribe glasses, contact lenses, low vision rehabilitation and medications
- Perform minor surgical procedures such as the removal of foreign bodies

An optometrist is a Doctor of Optometry or O.D.. This is not to be confused with a Doctor of Medicine, which is an M.D.. An optometrist must complete a pre-professional undergraduate college education and an additional four (4) years of professional education in a College of Optometry. Some optometrists also do a residency.

An ophthalmologist is an M.D. or a medical doctor who specializes in eye and vision care. Ophthalmologists are educated and trained to provide the full spectrum of eye care, from prescribing glasses and contact lenses to the most difficult and delicate eye surgeries.

Ophthalmologists must complete four (4) years of medical school, one year of rotating internships, and then a minimum of three years in residency in ophthalmology. A residency in ophthalmology concentrates and focuses on all aspects of eye care, including prevention, diagnosis and medical and surgical treatment of eye conditions and diseases. Ophthalmologists may also spend an additional year or two in residency to further specialize in more specialized areas of the eye such as the cornea, external disease, glaucoma, Neuro-Ophthalmology, Ophthalmic Pathology, Ophthalmic Plastic Surgery, Pediatric Ophthalmology, or Vitreoretinal diseases.

Question: Why have I not heard about the effectiveness of vision therapy?

Like most medical doctors, many optometrists and ophthalmologists follow the medical model of healing through medication, surgery, or prescription eyeglasses and will likely tell you that engaging in eyesight improvement programs or performing eye exercises to naturally improve eyesight can only be psychologically beneficial.

The reluctance of some doctors to try alternative methods of healing may cause one to ask whether their doctor truly has an interest in healing them or if they are simply treating and minimizing symptoms. Healing a patient completely increases the likelihood that many of their patients may not come back for their services. Fewer patient visits would likely result in reductions in office revenue.

In the defense of medical doctors, many are only taught the medical model of healing, or only one way of trying to heal a person, which is treating only the symptoms of a disorder and not the actual cause of the disorder.

For instance, eyeglasses and contact lenses do not improve eyesight; they merely balance visual defects by treating the symptoms of the problem, not the cause. Over months and years, wearing eyeglasses becomes habitual. Consequently, the original problem that caused the reduction in your vision quality persists, and may result in further deterioration of your visual acuity. As you lose more visual acuity, the strength of your correction, eyeglasses, or contacts, must increase or be adjusted. Your eyeglasses become one of the causes of blurry vision. As a result, you may regularly need stronger correction to see the same visual field clearly.

Internet searches will provide many different thoughts and statements about the "medical model" of vision treatment. One viewpoint of the medical model of healing was shared in an interview by Ms. Rachel Cooper of Optometrists Network of Leonard J. Press, FCOVD, FAAO who is the author of the textbook "Applied Concepts in Vision Therapy."[5] Ms. Cooper asked Dr. Press why some ophthalmologists and their organizations would claim that vision therapy does not work. Dr. Press provided the following statement:

"In 1993, Paul Romano, MD, the editor of Eye Muscle Surgery Quarterly, conducted a worldwide survey of eye muscle surgeons. He asked surgeons to indicate whether they would favor a surgical or non-surgical approach to the treatment of intermittent exotropia (a form of strabismus; a condition in which the eyes are not properly aligned with each other. It typically involves a lack of coordination between the extra ocular muscles, which prevents bringing the gaze of each eye to the same point in space, preventing proper binocular vision, which may adversely affect depth perception.). The results were that 85 percent of the international group recommended non surgical approaches, as compared with only 52 percent of the American surgeons. Dr. Romano postulated three important reasons why this might be so:

1. Insurance companies and single-payer systems outside of the U.S. have stricter medical standards in regards to approving payment of eye muscle surgery. Also, they do not pay as well for eye muscle surgery as insurance companies in the U.S.

2. Non surgical therapy isn't as economically rewarding for the surgeon in the U.S. due to the personnel and fees involved.

3. Due to his lack of training in this area, the surgeon is reluctant to acknowledge the benefits of non surgical therapy for fear of losing patients."

The full interview can be found at reference number 6.[6]

Dr. Romano's statement seems to indicate that there is a correlation between the type of treatment recommended and monetary compensation for that treatment by medical insurance companies.

Although Dr. Romano's statement is in response to treatment on intermittent exotropia, the issues he addressed are applicable to the ideologies of surgical treatment for other disorders and for the medical model of healing in general.

Chapter 3 About Eyesight

Statistics on the prevalence of vision problems

Estimates of those in the general population that need corrective lenses ranges from 75 to 90 percent, depending on the source consulted as well as the factors that are used for the criteria; these factors being age, sex, and the activities that the visual correction is needed for, such as reading or driving. According to the Vision Council of America in 2009, approximately 75 percent of adults used some sort of vision correction for blurred vision.[7] Statistics show that 64 percent of these people wear eyeglasses, and about 11 percent wear contact lenses, either exclusively, or with glasses. Over half of all women and about 42 percent of men wear eyeglasses.

Regardless of the accuracy of the total percentages, the drastic and continual increase in the number of adults that require visual correction for blurry vision is not disputed.

Improving Eyesight

There are three ways to improve eyesight and correct visual acuity; one is through correction such as eyeglasses or contact lenses, two is surgery, and three is vision therapy. These are discussed in more detail in Chapter 4.

Before considering any method or procedure to improve your visual acuity whether by correction, surgical, or natural means, it is important to understand how vision is possible, as well as the major factors that affect your visual acuity. Learning how your eyesight works will help you to better understand how you can naturally improve your eyesight.

How Does Your Eyesight Work?

The eye is an organ

The eye is an organ second in complexity only to the brain. The eye detects light and converts it into electro-chemical impulses that are interpreted by different parts of the brain. The simplest photoreceptor cells in the conscious vision of some organisms connect light to movement. In higher organisms like man, the eye is a complex optical system which collects light from the surrounding environment, regulates its intensity, focuses it through an adjustable lens assembly to form an image, chemically converts this image into a set of electrical signals, and transmits these signals through complex neural pathways via the optic nerve to the visual cortex and other areas of the brain. Problems that occur anywhere in this process can result in poor vision.

Light into sight

Light enters the eye and passes through the cornea where the lens focuses the light onto the retina. The retina is part of the central nervous system; it originates from developing brain tissue so it is considered to be part of the brain. The retina contains two types of cells called rods and cones. The cones determine color vision and detail, and the rods determine vision in low light. When light makes contact with either of these two types of cells, a series of complex chemical reactions takes place. These chemicals produce electrical impulses that when transmitted to the visual cortex of the brain, are interpreted as the objects you "see". The chemicals used to create electrical impulses are derived from vitamin A, which is why vitamin A deficiencies result in vision problems.

Parts of the Eye

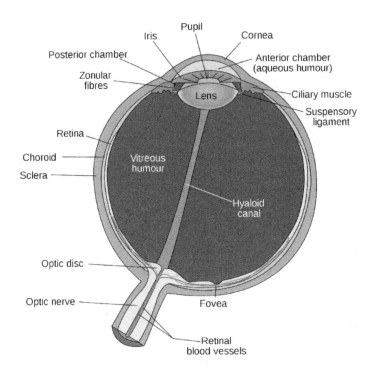

Learning the structure of the eye helps one to understand how eyesight works.

- The <u>sclera</u>, the outermost layer of the eye, is partially visible as the "white" of the eye. It maintains the shape of the eye.

- At the front of the eye projecting slightly, is the <u>cornea</u>. It is completely clear transparent membrane that acts as the window of the eye. It also provides approximately two thirds of the optical power of the eye. All light must first pass through the cornea when it enters the eye. The shape of the cornea is fixed; it does not change its shape to focus the optical system. The cornea does not have any blood supply to provide oxygen or nutrients. Oxygen dissolves in the tears and diffuses throughout the cornea. Nutrients are provided by the aqueous humor, a transparent gelatinous fluid secreted by the ciliary processes, the structure that supports the lens.

- The choroid, the layer beneath the sclera, is composed of dense pigment and blood vessels that supply blood to the eye. Near the center of the visible part of the eye, the choroid forms the ciliary body.

- The ciliary muscle is attached to the lens, and contracts and relaxes to control the shape and size of the lens to provide variable focusing. There are three sets of ciliary muscles in the eye, the longitudinal, radial, and circular muscles. They are near the front of the eye, above and below the lens.

- The ciliary body is composed of the ciliary muscle and ciliary processes that includes the choroid. The ciliary processes produce the aqueous humor, the transparent gelatinous fluid that provides nutrients to the cornea.

- The iris is a muscular diaphragm that adjusts and regulates the size of the pupil. The iris gives the eye its color by revealing the choroid's pigmentation. The most common eye colors are brown or blue.

- The pupil is the round opening through which light enters the eye. The iris and pupil have a set of muscles that control the opening of the pupil and the amount of light that is allowed into the eye.

- Behind the iris is the <u>lens</u> which is a transparent, elastic, but solid ellipsoid body that with the cornea bends light rays focusing them on the retina. The lens is a clear dual convex structure that changes shape based on the contractions of the ciliary muscles. The ciliary muscles adjust the shape of the lens to perfect visual acuity.

- <u>Zonule of Zinn or zonular fibers</u> are a ring of fibrous strands that connect the ciliary body to the lens. The fibers attach around the edges of the lens and it is theorized that they assist the lens in flattening out when the ciliary muscles relax.

- At the back of the eye is the <u>retina</u>, which contains the network of nerve cells called rods and cones that chemically react to light waves to create the electrical impulses that travel along the optic nerve to other parts of the brain. Rods allow you to see objects in dim light; the cones work the best in bright light and determine colors. The retina contains a chemical called rhodopsin that converts light into electrical impulses sent through the optic nerve that the brain interprets as vision. The retina is brain tissue and considered to be part of the brain.

Visual Perception

Visual perception is the ability to interpret the surrounding environment by processing information contained in visible light. The resulting perception is also known as eyesight, sight, or vision. The various physiological components involved in vision are referred to collectively as the visual system.

The Visual System

The visual system in man allows for the assimilation of information from the environment. Man's visual system is a complex optical system. Most complex optical systems have several movable lens assemblies in order to be capable of producing variable focus. The optical system in man contains the cornea which is a non adjustable lens responsible for approximately two thirds of the optical power of the eye. The optical system also contains the lens which is the only part of the eye that provides adjustable optical power.

An optical lens is simply a smooth, curved transparent substance; it is called convex if curved outward like the outside of a ball, and concave if curved inward like the inside of a bowl. The curved surface of the lens in man is convex or rounded, being thicker in the middle and thinner at the edges.

The center of any lens is called the center of curvature. All rays of light passing through a lens are refracted or bent except for those that pass directly through the center of curvature. The center of curvature of any lens is also called the optical center.

A concave or divergent lens, or one that is thicker at the edges than at the center, bends light rays that are parallel to the axis of the lens away from each other. The image formed by a diverging lens is always erect (upright), smaller than the object, and virtual (located on the same side of the lens as the object).

A convex or convergent lens, or one that is thicker at the center than at the edges, bends parallel light rays toward one another. If the light rays entering the lens are parallel to the principal axis of the lens, they converge to a common point, or focus, behind the lens. The proper focus of an image formed by a converging lens is dependent on the distance of the object in relation to the lens's focal length and its center of curvature. In the eye of man, the focal length is the distance between the center of the lens and the principal point of focus on the retina. To keep the focus of an image consistent and sharp at a constant focal length, the shape of the lens must change as the distance of the object being viewed changes.

The ciliary muscles change the shape of the lens by constricting or relaxing in order to maintain clear image focus on the retina at the constant given focal length based on the varying distance of the object that is to be "seen" or focused on. The ciliary muscles change the shape of the lens to control the convergence of light waves and where the light waves are focused on the retina. Optical power is possible because the ciliary muscles change the shape of the elastic lens, either by squeezing the lens or by relaxing and allowing the lens to expand. When the ciliary muscles constrict the lens it thickens, increasing optical power. When the ciliary muscles relax, the lens flattens out with the help of zonular fibers that connect to the lens around the edges holding it in the proper position.

A convergent lens inverts images, turning them upside down. As the lens in the eye of man is a convergent lens, the brain must rectify the inverted images that are created by the lens.

The act of "seeing" starts when the lens in the eye focuses the light reflected off of an image onto the light-sensitive membrane in the back of the eye, called the retina. The retina is a part of the brain that is isolated to serve as a transducer for the conversion of patterns of light into neuronal signals. When the lens focuses light on the retina, the photoreceptive cells detect and react to the photons in the light waves. The photons initiate chemical reactions in these cells that produce electrical neural impulses. The retina sends the electrical impulses along the optic nerve to the visual cortex of the brain. These signals are processed in a hierarchical fashion by different parts of the brain, from the retina to the central ganglia located in the brain and are then decoded or deciphered as the particular images that the light waves reflected off.

An eye with either too much or too little refractive power that does not focus light at the right place on the retina has a refractive error. Either of these conditions reduces visual acuity. A myopic or nearsighted eye has too much power, so light is focused too much in front of the retina. Conversely, a hyperopic or farsighted eye has too little power and light is focused too far behind the retina. A hyperopic eye occurs when the lens is too flat and cannot be constricted into enough of a rounded shape.

Most of the time when there is a problem with visual acuity, eye doctors "correct" the problem by prescribing an additional corrective lens that is to be placed in front of the eye in either an eyeglass frame or as a contact lens. Adding a lens to the visual system makes an adjustment in the focal length between the lens and retina. Given a set focal point, the additional lens changes the point on the retina that the light rays are focused at.

Visual Acuity

Visual acuity is the clearness of vision or the ability to distinguish fine detail. It is the function of the cone cells in the retina to differentiate between the different visual angles and depths of various light rays.

The eye contains multiple transparent angulated surfaces that cause light waves to bend. When the visual system is working properly, the light waves arrive in perfect focus at the right spot on the retina for interpretation, resulting in clear vision. When light rays are not focused at the right location on the retina, a reduction in visual acuity or blurry vision results.

Errors in properly transferring chemical and/or electrical signals or in the brain's ability to interpret electrical signals of properly focused light can also result in vision problems.

Accommodation

Accommodation describes the process of the optical system in adjusting the lens for variable optical power in order to maintain clear focus of objects at different distances or as an object's distance changes. Accommodation requires the shape of the lens to change to maintain clear focus on an object based on the object's effective distance. Accommodation normally happens automatically, as a reflex, _but it can also be consciously controlled_. We can change the optical power of our visual system by using the ciliary muscle to change the shape of the elastic lens.

Unfortunately, accommodation in the visual system can decline with age. Once this process starts, the decline can either happen slowly or rather quickly without some type of intervention.

The ability to consciously control and affect accommodation is an important element of vision therapy.

Factors That Affect Visual Acuity

From a technical standpoint, visual acuity is limited by diffraction, optical aberrations, and photoreceptor density in the eye. These are things that you cannot correct. Apart from these limitations, there are a number of factors that affect visual acuity that can be influenced, such as refractive error, illumination, contrast, and the location on the retina that is being stimulated. The focus of the lens can adjust to the changing shape of the eyeball, light can be controlled in some situations, contrast can be changed on electronic screens, special text can be chosen for increased contrast, and the shape of the lens determines where light is focused on the retina.

Besides the impacts of disease and certain types of medications, there are three (3) main factors that impact visual acuity and cause blurry vision:

1. Use of Visual range

Before technology and modern life brought most people indoors and required them to work for long periods of time at close distances, we "exercised" our eyes naturally. While outdoors or not confined to places that limit our viewing ranges, we exercised our eyes and kept our visual acuity sharp by continuously varying the distances we focused our vision at.

The full use of all of our visual ranges regularly throughout the day is very important. Although the eye doctors who prescribe corrective lenses may disagree with the following analogy, it might be helpful to further one's understanding. Limiting visual ranges might be compared to limiting the range of motion that your arm may bend at the elbow or your leg may bend at the knee. While using either appendage in a drastically limited range for the majority of time that the appendage is used, for periods of weeks or years, one could not expect the appendage to function at full capacity and strength when it is used in its full range of motion. The muscles and supporting connective tissues that are responsible for proper operation would not be maintained in the condition necessary to function at 100 percent. When we do not use a full range of motion the body responds by allowing the affected areas to become weaker. Anyone who has worn a cast for a short period of only a few weeks is fully aware of what effect immobility has on muscles as well as the related supporting and connective tissues. Those who have had an injured limb immobilized for any length of time understand that the affected areas become weaker as a result of not being fully utilized.

Fully utilizing all ranges of your visual system naturally exercises the variable focus of your complex optical system.

Variable focusing at long distances: To focus on objects at greater distances, the ciliary muscle must relax around the lens in order to allow the lens to flatten out, become thinner and wider increasing lens diameter and decreasing magnifying power. As muscles only constrict, the ciliary muscle can only tighten around the lens to decrease its diameter making it thicker and increasing magnifying power. When the ciliary muscle relaxes, the lens must be elastic enough to flatten out and assume its normal un-flexed shape, either on its own or with the help of the supportive connecting zonular fibers. Some doctors theorize that the zonular fibers which attach around the outside of the lens help the lens to flatten out by stretching it out or pulling it into a flattened position. Whether this is true or not, in some cases the lens does not flatten out which causes problems in the optical system for focusing clearly at greater distances. When the visual system is working properly, the lens flattens out increasing in diameter and decreasing the magnification power in the eye to change the focal point on the retina just enough to balance out the distance of the object being focused on. It is important to focus on objects at longer distances regularly throughout the day to allow the lens to flatten out. Without periodically relaxing the ciliary muscles around the lens, the flexibility of the lens can be lost over time.

Variable focusing at short distances: To focus on objects at close distances, the ciliary muscle must tighten around the lens in order to make the lens thicker, decreasing the diameter and increasing magnifying power. When the ciliary muscle tightens, the lens must flexible enough to be placed into a thicker shape that is more rounded, closer to the shape of a ball. The ciliary muscle must be able to squeeze the lens into the proper corresponding thicker and more rounded shape in order to place the focal point at the right place on the retina. When the visual system is working properly, the lens decreases in diameter and moves into the just the right thickness to increase the magnification power enough to keep the focal point at the right location on the retina to balance out the closer distance of the object you are trying to see. This normally happens automatically as a reflex, but in some cases the lens does not increase to the right thickness which prevents the optical system from focusing clearly at close distances. It is important to focus on objects at close distances regularly throughout the day to keep the ciliary muscles properly calibrated and strong enough to squeeze the lens into the right shape, and also to maintain lens elasticity. Without periodically tightening the ciliary muscles around the lens to change the shape of the lens throughout the day, the flexibility of the lens over time can diminish. When lens elasticity is lost, it becomes much harder for the ciliary muscle to squeeze the rigid lens into the correct shape to focus at close ranges. Focusing on objects up close regularly throughout the day can help the keep the lens from losing its flexibility as one ages.

Be sure to focus on objects at varying distances in your visual range throughout the day to naturally exercise your eyes and to keep your focus sharp and calibrated at all distances. Fully utilizing all of the ranges of your visual system regularly throughout the day naturally exercises the variable focus of your complex optical system and helps to relieve accumulated eye strain.

2. Accumulated Stress and Tension

Accumulated stress and tension in the eye or the body can affect visual acuity.

The body is a remarkable machine that readily adapts to stress. Stress can affect your body in either positive or negative ways based on the type of stress and amount of stress that is experienced. Additional stress demands on the body can cause it to grow stronger; the lack of stress can cause it to weaken. The body adapts to most reasonable amounts of stress by strengthening itself and the affected areas. For instance, some mental stress can force us to handle that stress better by desensitizing our reaction to it or by motivating us to take action to mitigate it, such as learning and changing our behavior. One result could be becoming more organized and efficient by prioritizing tasks and utilizing our available time better. Your body reacts to stress from appropriate amounts of weight lifting exercises by strengthening muscles, bones, and connective tissues. Too much mental stress can cause an overload that can shut down cognitive processes and increase stress related hormones like cortisol. If one engages in too much weight lifting, the muscles and connective tissues can become overworked and inflamed, and pull or strain. The prolonged excessive use of overworked muscles and tissues in the body can result in an accumulation of inflammation in those particular muscles and tissues that in time, can weaken and severely limit their functioning, as well as increase overall body cortisol levels.

Focusing the visual system throughout its full ocular range regularly throughout the day is a good stress that strengthens and helps to keep the focusing power of the visual system sharp and calibrated. Stress that accumulates in the eye becomes eye strain; this is bad stress, and it has a negative impact on your vision. Utilizing the full viewing range regularly throughout the day is one way that the eye naturally relieves accumulated stress.

Because ciliary muscles must relax or loosen their constriction of the lens to allow for focusing at greater distances, accumulated eye strain is not usually associated with focusing at long distances. Stress is not likely to accumulate in the eye when attempting to focus at longer ranges. While one may have difficulty viewing objects clearly at longer distances or at the further points of their optical range, the struggle is to relax the ciliary muscles and lens tissue to get the lens to flatten out.

In order to focus on objects up close, the ciliary muscle must contract around the lens to make it thicker. To maintain focus on objects or images at close distances, the ciliary muscle must stay tightly contracted around the lens and keep it balled up to sustain the focal point at the proper location on the retina. Keeping the ciliary muscles tightened around the lens to sustain focus on objects at close distances for long periods of time can cause stress and eye strain to build up in the ciliary muscles, lens, and surrounding tissues. When the lens is held tightly in a balled up position for long periods of time, day after day for months or years, stress and strain may continue to accumulate in the ciliary muscle, lens and surrounding structures and affect their ability to work together to perform properly. The ciliary muscle can have difficulty relaxing to allow the lens to increase in diameter and the elasticity of the lens can be lost which can inhibit it from being able to flatten out properly to focus at longer ranges.

In these modern times, both life and work has brought most people indoors causing them to spend long periods of time focusing at close distances. Office work may require staring at computer screens for long periods of time. Students and those in many professional occupations may spend many hours or a majority of their time daily staring at computer screens, reading books, writing documents or performing other activities at close distances.

Just as stress can affect other parts of the body, accumulated eye strain from focusing up close for long periods of time can negatively affect the ability of the ciliary muscle to place the lens into the right shape to focus light at the right location on the retina. Keeping the lens tightly constricted can cause the lens to lose elasticity and the ability to flatten out. Either of these conditions or the combination of both of them can prevent the visual system from functioning as necessary to properly focus light waves at the correct spot on the retina for clear image interpretation.

Certain visual practices can create a considerable amount of eye strain in the ciliary muscle and lens. Visual practices like reading, writing, viewing computer screens, watching television, or any other activity that requires focusing at close distances for long periods of time without taking appropriate breaks can produce stress and strain that can accumulate in the optical system and affect visual acuity. Operating your optical system at close distances indoors or by staring at electronic devices like a computer screen, e-reader, or cell phone can cause computer vision syndrome. The term computer vision syndrome refers to a group of eye and vision-related symptoms that result from prolonged computer use and will be discussed in more detail in following chapters.

Those who read, study, view computer screens, or otherwise focus at very close ranges for long periods of time may notice that when they look away from what they are doing at close distances to longer distances, they have difficulty focusing clearly on objects at the longer distances. The exact range of these longer distances may vary based on a number of factors such as time and frequency of the close range focusing, but visual acuity could be affected by looking only as far as the other side of a normal sized room. If one had the ability to focus clearly at the longer distance that is now blurry prior to engaging in the close focus activity, the ability to regain clear focus on images at the longer distances usually returns in a short period of time once the accumulated eye strain has been relieved and the lens is able to flatten out. Cessation of close distance focus and shifting focus to longer distances usually helps to relieve the accumulated strain more quickly. Those who continue to focus at very close distances without taking breaks to relieve eye strain may notice that the described condition occurs more often, increases in severity, or that it takes a longer time for normal vision acuity to return, if it does at all. Many times those who experience this condition may not notice that normal visual acuity does not return completely.

Accumulated eye strain from visual practices can be the sole cause of poor visual acuity and blurry vision. Visual acuity is greatly affected by eye strain and the quality of your vision can gradually diminish as eye strain accumulates. At first, you may only notice temporary blurred vision for short time periods of time or when shifting your focus from near to far distances, particularly after performing activities that require close distance focus. Although blurred vision may not initially be as noticeable, it will likely become more apparent as the quality of vision deteriorates and becomes more blurry or the condition occurs more often. This condition helps many to understand why those who once had normal 20/20 or better vision are now myopic and need corrective lenses. Myopia, or nearsightedness, is the most common eye condition needing correction among young people.[8] The American Optometric Association estimates that up to 30 percent of the entire American population including all ages, suffer from nearsightedness.

Poor visual acuity can contribute to or be the sole cause of a multitude of other problems such as headaches, slower reading speeds, and the inability to concentrate.

With respect to eye stress from visual practices, the limiting of your visual range to short distances for substantial portions of the day repetitively without taking the necessary breaks can cause eye strain to accumulate over time which is likely to decrease your ability to focus at further distances. More information on how to take breaks while reading, studying, or viewing computer screens as well as ways to use vision therapy to reduce eye stress from these practices will be discussed in more detail in following chapters.

Visual acuity is not only affected by stress that originates from visual practices. The fast pace of life and often unreasonable amounts of stress resulting from work, children, relationships, or other life events create stress in both the mind and body. Stress and tension in the body has been shown to have a pronounced effect on mental operations, physical condition, and visual acuity.

The eyes are most affected by muscle stress in the upper body. Visual acuity is largely affected by stress in the face, jaw, neck, and shoulders. Some doctors maintain that correlations have been established linking stress in specific areas of the body to specific eyesight problems. Nearsighted people tend to have chronic muscle stress in the shoulders and neck, while farsighted people tend to have chronic stress in the face, jaw, and throat areas. Research indicates that overall stress relief and relaxation is important for good visual acuity.

It is well understood and accepted, even in medical circles, that mental stress can cause physical symptoms and ailments. Unhealthy levels of mental stress or the inability to manage stress levels can have a substantial impact on the body's hormonal production, and a deteriorating affect on visual acuity and health. The lack of sleep can increase levels of stress and affect visual acuity. Emotional distress, no matter the cause, can affect visual acuity. Stress can inhibit accommodation in the visual system. Poor accommodation reduces visually acuity and can lead to other problems such as nearsightedness, farsightedness, or other visual disorders.

The effects of stress on visual acuity were well researched and documented as early as 1920 by William Horatio Bates, who was referenced in Chapter 2. Dr. Bate's research linked visual acuity with stress. When we are relaxed and healthy we see at our best, if we are tired, tense, or ill, we see at our worst. If stress is relieved, eyesight will improve. Eyesight can deteriorate or improve rapidly or slowly. Over time Dr. Bates found that accumulated stress causes the ciliary muscles to weaken which can alter the focal point in your eye and reduce accommodation.[9]

High levels of tension in the body will decrease the synthesis and utilization of helpful hormones and increase the body's production of stress related hormones such as cortisol. High levels of cortisol have been proven through scientific studies relating to Cushing's Disease or Cushing's Syndrome to speed the aging process and over time, negatively affect all tissues in the body.[10]

With respect to accumulated stress and tension, either eye strain or physical and mental stresses are enough to noticeably decrease visual acuity independent of each other let alone in combination. Vision therapy relieves accumulated eye stress. To get the greatest benefit from vision therapy you should also seek to reduce and control physical and mental stress. Stress relief is covered more in the following chapters.

3. Aging

Aging can be a cause of visual deterioration. Aging can affect the regeneration and repair of eye tissue that is directly responsible for visual acuity and alter conditions in body that can substantially impact the onset of eye disease and general physical disease.

Other than the impact of disease and certain types of medication, the use of visual range, accumulated tension, and aging are the main factors that affect visual acuity and are the primary causes of blurry vision.

Why Does Eyesight Worsen as We Age?

As we age, the cells in our body lose their ability to regenerate.

Aging can cause the ciliary muscle to become weak and supportive tissues to lose elasticity. When the lens becomes less elastic and loses its ability to change shape, a condition called Presbyopia results. Those affected with this condition have difficulty focusing on or are not able to focus on objects that are at close distances. As the lens loses flexibility, the ciliary muscles must work harder to contract around the lens to squeeze it into a thicker shape. The accumulated strain in the ciliary muscle and loss of lens elasticity affects the ability of the lens to change shape to become thicker to properly focus on close objects.

Those with inflexible lenses that are not able to flatten out are forced to hold objects farther away from their eyes in order to focus on them clearly. In many of those that are affected, this condition becomes more noticeable in the age range of the mid-forties. If the elasticity of the lens continues to decrease, the lens will be unable to flex much at all and can become more or less permanently focused at a fixed distance, which can be different for each person affected.

Preventing the negative effects of aging is the subject of Chapter 5.

Common Conditions that Affect the Quality of Vision

Nearsightedness or myopia is a condition where a person is able to see near objects well but has difficulty seeing objects that are far away. This is because the lens is focusing light rays too far in front of the retina. It is caused by a lens system that is focusing the eye with too much power or an eyeball that is too long. Nearsightedness can be corrected by using less lens power to focus light. Nearsightedness is more common than farsightedness in young people and there is growing evidence to support that it is influenced by visual practices such as focusing at close distances for extended periods of time. Recent statistics from AOA estimate that up to 30 percent of the American population suffers from nearsightedness (American Optometric Association).

Farsightedness or hyperopia is a condition where a person is able to see distant objects well and has difficulty seeing objects that are near. This is because the lens is focusing light rays too far behind the retina. It is caused by a lens system that will not thicken enough and is focusing the eye with too little focusing power, or by an eyeball that is too short. Farsightedness can be corrected by using more lens power to focus light. At younger ages, farsightedness is usually caused by heredity. At older ages farsightedness is usually caused by presbyopia. The Vision Council of America estimates that about 60 percent of Americans are far-sighted meaning they have trouble reading or sewing without glasses, but can focus well at a distance.[11]

Common Eye Diseases

Astigmatism is an optical defect where objects cannot be properly focused on the retina because of the uneven curvature of the cornea or the shape of the lens which prevents proper focus of light waves on the retina. This can occur in combination with other vision conditions such as nearsightedness or farsightedness. This condition is usually present in some degree in most people. Medical treatments include eyeglasses, contact lenses, or surgery. If you have this condition vision therapy can help to adjust the focal point of the lens to improve visual acuity.

Cataracts result from a cloudiness in the lens that blocks light from reaching the retina. Loss in vision acuity occurs because the cloudiness prevents light from passing through the lens to be focused at the right location on the retina. The most common cause of cataracts is aging. Cigarette smoking increases the risk of cataracts. Some medication such as corticosteroids increase the risk of cataracts. Cataracts are the most common cause of blindness. Anti-aging protocols including proper diet, nutrition, not smoking, physical exercise, and stress relief can help prevent cataracts. Surgery is also used to remove cataracts. Those with cataracts may be able to see better with pinhole glasses. Vision therapy can help to better focus the light waves that make it through the cornea and lens.

Presbyopia is a condition where the lens of the eye loses its flexibility making it difficult to focus on close objects. The condition may seem to occur suddenly, but the loss of flexibility usually takes place over a number of years. This condition usually becomes noticeable in the age range of early to mid forties. Presbyopia is reported by the medical industry to be a natural part of the aging process that cannot be prevented. Signs of presence of this condition include holding reading materials at arm's length, blurred vision at normal reading distance and eye fatigue along with headaches when doing close work.

Glaucoma is a condition where the eye fluid or aqueous humor does not properly drain out of the eye which causes intraocular pressure to build up in the eye. The increase in pressure can cause the cells and nerve fibers in the back of the eye to die. Certain types of medication such as prolonged use of steroids can cause glaucoma. Severely restricted blood flow to the eyes can cause glaucoma. Anti-aging protocols including proper diet, nutrition, physical exercise, and stress relief can help prevent glaucoma. Medical treatments include medication and/or surgery can be effective.

Diabetic retinopathy: Usually those with diabetes are more likely to have blockage of blood vessels or leakage of blood vessels that can cause scarring or damage to the retina that can eventually lead to blindness. After the diagnosis of diabetes, chances of developing diabetic retinopathy increase over time. Controlling diabetes and blood sugar through proper diet and nutrition can help prevent diabetic retinopathy. Laser surgery and injection of corticosteroids are other treatments used for diabetic retinopathy.

Macular degeneration The macula is an oval shaped area near the center of the retina about 5.5 millimeters in size. As some people age, the macula which is responsible for fine detail in the retina for the center of vision, can deteriorate for unknown reasons. This condition causes loss of central vision. Age Related Eye Disease Study (AREDS) trials have found benefits from the use of vitamin and mineral supplements and high doses of antioxidants in both the prevention and treatment of macular degeneration. Those afflicted with macular degeneration can better learn to use their peripheral vision for eyesight.

There are many causes of blindness; vitamin A deficiency, toxins, infections, strokes, neurological diseases, and hereditary diseases.

Vision therapy is not intended to completely replace your eye doctor. If you are experiencing problems with your vision, it is important to be diagnosed by an eye doctor to eliminate the possibility of eye disease.

Chapter 4 About Vision Therapy Programs

This chapter addresses the three ways eyesight can be improved, improving visual acuity and correcting visual practices, and how corrective lenses harm eyesight. The sections; what makes an effective vision therapy program, computer vision syndrome, and pinhole glasses, follow.

Three Ways Eyesight can be Improved

There are three ways to improve visual acuity:

1. Lens correction, such as eyeglasses or contact lenses
2. Surgery
3. Vision therapy

Lens Correction

Eyeglasses and contact lenses improve visual acuity in the visual system by changing or adjusting the lens point of focus on the retina. While eyeglasses and contact lenses may increase visual acuity for a certain undefined period of time, this type of correction does not address the underlying cause of the visual problem.

Blurry vision could be caused by a number of things including the size and length of your eyeball, the clarity and evenness of the cornea, as well as the elasticity of the lens and the strength and calibration of the ciliary muscle. These can all change over time.

Medical research supports that the size and length of your eyeball can fluctuate. Changes in the length of the eyeball can change the eye's focal length. Many conditions such as infection or allergies can affect the evenness of the cornea. Aging and the amount of close distance focusing can affect the elasticity of the lens and the calibration of the ciliary muscle.

The shape of the lens determines the focal point on the retina. The ciliary muscle must be able to make fine adjustments in the shape of the lens to place the focal point of the object you are viewing at the proper place on the retina in relation to the focal length in order for you to see it clearly. Correcting visual acuity with eyeglasses or contact lenses does not permanently address any of the listed conditions; it serves only as a temporary fix. Those with eyeglasses or contact lenses often find that their prescription needs to change and the strength must be increased.

Surgery

Eye surgery such as LASIK or PRK, may increase visual acuity in some areas of vision for an undefined period of time but neither permanently address the cause of poor visual acuity.

Eye surgery to improve visual acuity can have complications in some specific areas of visual acuity such as; glare, the appearance of halos around images and lights, poor night vision, dry eyes, and can result in post surgery vision that is not entirely clear at all distances.

If eye disease is present, eye surgery may be necessary and the best available option.

Vision Therapy

Vision therapy works to naturally improve eyesight by strengthening the ciliary muscles of the eye, promoting the flexibility of the lens, relieving eye strain, and calibrating the focal point on the retina. Vision therapy strengthens the visual system and sharpens visual acuity. For all vision problems that can be corrected with eye glasses or contact lenses, the sole cause of the visual problem is the inability of the lens to focus light waves at the proper point on the retina. Vision therapy can help to correct these problems.

Vision therapy relieves temporary and accumulated stress on the ciliary muscles of the eye. Vision therapy strengthens the ciliary muscles in the eye and helps maintain lens elasticity. Vision therapy helps to calibrate the focal point in the eye and coordinate both eyes working together. Vision therapy can even help to improve the visual acuity of those with vision problems caused by eye disease. The benefit of performing vision therapy is well documented. There are many testimonials to the helpful benefits of vision therapy.

Nearly all who engage in vision therapy will see immediate improvements in the quality of their vision and abilities of accommodation. Keep in mind that any deterioration or change in accommodation that reduced visual acuity likely did not occur overnight; therefore all who utilize vision therapy should not expect to see substantial improvements in the quality of vision immediately. Although the rate of improvement of those engaging in vision therapy may vary, progress is usually seen very early in the vision therapy program by all, usually in the very first therapy session.

Even though countless testimonials speak to the positive effects of vision therapy on the improvement and restoration of vision damaged from diseases such as astigmatism, glaucoma, and cataracts, it is important to understand that these exercises are not a miracle cure. It can sometimes take months of exercise before vision will improve, if it improves at all. Some damaged eyesight may never become 20/20 or better, even if vision therapy sessions were used many times per day, every day, for years. Even though your visual acuity may never improve to the point of discarding your corrective visual devices, it is still possible for it to increase and cease to deteriorate. Vision therapy itself is very relaxing to both the eye and the body. There is a very high probability that vision therapy will improve the visual acuity of your vision system.

Improving Visual Acuity and Correcting Visual Practices

If your visual acuity has deteriorated in the absence of disease, it has likely done so because of a decrease in the accommodation abilities of your visual system. The decrease in the accommodation abilities of your visual system could be due to a number of reasons as described in Chapter 3, "Factors That Affect Your Visual Acuity."

As covered in Chapter 3, ciliary muscles can become weak and lose calibration from not being "exercised" or focused throughout their full range of view. To help prevent this, be sure to focus on objects at varying distances in your visual range throughout the day to naturally exercise your eyes and keep your visual acuity sharp at all distances. Fully utilizing all of the ranges of your visual system regularly throughout the day exercises the variable focus of your complex optical system and naturally relieves accumulated eye strain in the ciliary muscle and lens. Do not maintain close focusing for extended periods of time without taking appropriate breaks. It has been theorized that the amount of focusing you perform daily at short or long distances can affect the shape of the eyeball. For instance when you focus for long periods of time at close distances your eyeball will elongate making it easier for you to focus clearly for longer periods of time at close distances. The elongation of the eyeball can make it harder for you to focus at longer distances. If you have blurry vision at a particular range or distance, you should target that range more frequently in vision therapy.

As stated in Chapter 3, stress can have a substantial impact on visual acuity. With respect to accumulated stress and tension, either eye strain or physical and mental stresses can noticeably decrease visual acuity independent of each other, let alone in combination. Use vision therapy to relieve accumulated eye stress. To get the greatest benefit from vision therapy you should also seek to relieve as much physical and mental stress as possible.

There are many ways to relieve physical and mental stress. A physical exercise program will help to relieve physical and mental stress. Getting enough sleep will help to relieve physical and mental stress. Visual acuity can be significantly affected by the amount of sleep that you get. Massage therapy or chiropractic adjustments may also provide significant reductions in stress as well as an increase in overall heath and well being.

Stress can affect the shape of the eyeball. The shape of the eyeball can affect vision by changing the focal length in the eye. Research indicates that the eyeball's shape is not fixed and can change in response to many factors such as stress, disease, and the effects of aging. These temporary fluctuations in the shape of the eye can affect visual acuity. It has been proposed that the shape and length of the eye can fluctuate back and forth based solely on stress levels. Dr. Bates and the related work of other physician's indicates that conditions of nearsightedness and farsightedness are not permanent conditions, they are affected by the shape of the eyeball, and that the shape of the eyeball can change as we age and in response to stress. In a normal healthy visual system absent of any contributing visual problems, the ciliary muscles would fine tune the lens shape and focal point to compensate for a slightly different focal length and clear vision would be maintained.

It is highly recommended that you follow a program of overall stress reduction. Stress reduction is addressed in more detail in Chapter 5.

As covered in Chapter 3, aging can be a cause of visual deterioration. Aging affects the regeneration and repair of tissues in the eye as well as the onset of eye disease and general physical disease. The negative effects of aging can be delayed or reversed by proper diet and nutrition and activities such as physical exercise and stress control that promote proper hormone secretion.

Combining different types of anaerobic and aerobic physical exercise results in an increase in the production and utilization of hormones that help to prevent and reverse the negative effects of aging. Proper hormone utilization is critical in controlling and reversing the effects of aging on the body and eyesight. Poor hormone optimization speeds the effects of aging and increases the likelihood of poor health, blurry vision and other potential negative effects on visual acuity.

Diet and nutrition are probably the single most important factors influencing the aging process. Proper diet and nutrition do not solely consist of consuming healthy foods. The elimination of certain foods and chemical food additives, the combination of proper types of foods, the amounts consumed, and the timing in which they are consumed have a huge impact on your health, the body's production and utilization of hormones, and the aging process. Improper nutrition is the leading cause of disease in the body.

When the accelerated effects of aging are combined with poor visual practices, there can be exponential negative effects on the visual system and substantial decreases in visual acuity.

Preventing the negative effects of aging is addressed further in Chapter 5.

Having a good understanding of how eyesight works and how certain visual practices affect eyesight is important to understand how good vision can deteriorate.

Nearsightedness is a condition where far objects appear blurred, but near objects are seen clearly. This condition can result from either the elongation of the eye from front to back or the ciliary muscles not releasing their tension around the lens or lens elasticity not allowing lens diameter to increase. Because the eyeball is too long or the eye's refractive power too strong, the image is focused in front of the retina of the eye. Eyeglasses with concave or divergent lenses are used to correct this condition.

Farsightedness is a condition when far objects can be seen clearly, but near objects appear blurry. This condition can result from either the shortening of the eye from front to back or the ciliary muscles not constricting the lens enough or lens elasticity not allowing lens diameter to decrease. Because the eyeball is too short, or the refractive power of the lens being too weak, an image is focused behind the retina of the eye. Eyeglasses with convex or convergent lenses are used to correct this condition.

Temporary disruptions in visual acuity caused by poor visual practices can become chronic and relatively permanent. Focusing at close distances for extended periods of time without taking proper breaks can cause strain in the ciliary muscle and in the lens keeping it from flattening out when the ciliary muscle is relaxed. Strain can accumulate when the ciliary muscle holds the lens in a balled up position for lengthy periods. Again, this muscle is not unlike other muscles in the body; it can become overworked and is negatively affected by accumulated strain and inflammation. The ciliary muscles can become tight and rigid from holding the lens in a fixed position for extended periods of time. The lens, being held in a tight balled up position can lose its flexibility. Lens elasticity is necessary to be able to focus clearly at long distances. When the lens is held tightly for long periods, it can take time for the lens to flatten out. When the lens has been held tightly for long periods, the ciliary muscles can struggle to relax and release the lens. The lens tissue has to relax and flatten out in order for you to focus clearly on objects at farther distances. As muscles can only contract, the ciliary muscle must relax for the lens to flatten out.

Improper visual practices such as reading without taking breaks are very stressful on the eyes; more specifically on the ciliary muscles and lens. Repeated strain from poor visual practices can accumulate and weaken the ciliary muscles affecting their abilities to focus the lens properly and contribute to lens loss of elasticity. As previously mentioned, those who have read for long periods of time at close distances without taking breaks have likely experienced mild or severe visual blurriness and possibly eye soreness. Blurry vision is more likely to be experienced when the text being read is held at close distances to the eyes. In mild cases, the visual blurriness might remain unnoticed until the person who has been reading looks away from the material being read, and attempts to focus on an object at a distance. Cases increasing in severity can result in blurry vision looking across the room where vision is normally clear. In more severe cases, eye pain, discomfort, and/or headaches can result and longer periods of time are necessary for normal clear vision to return.

Temporary visual impairment from close focusing or reading for extended periods can be alleviated by relaxing the ciliary muscles and allowing the lens to flatten out at regular intervals. The intervals necessary will be different for each person and will need to be determined by each person through experimentation. For many people, 30-90 second vision therapy breaks taken every 15 minutes may be needed. Eye strain can usually be relieved where vision returns to normal or close to normal in 10-

15 minutes after cessation of close distance focusing and upon shifting your focus from near to far distances, depending on the length of time close focus has been maintained. The longer the period of close focus, the longer it may take for clear vision to return. If focusing at close distances is a continual practice and consistently performed for long periods of time over the course of months or years without relieving any accumulated eye strain, visual acuity can be negatively affected to the point that it may not return to normal without some type of intervention such as vision therapy. As stress accumulates in the ciliary muscle affecting its calibration and the lens slowly loses its elasticity, any deterioration in visual acuity may not be noticeable at first. As the ciliary muscle becomes more strained and the lens loses more elasticity, they can become less calibrated as a team and it becomes harder for them to work together to maintain visual acuity.

To prevent visual impairment from close focusing or reading for extended periods of time follow the 20-20-20 rule. The 20-20-20 rule calls for one to look away from the screen at an object that is at least 20 feet away, every 20 minutes, for 20 seconds. Vision therapy exercises can be performed during these short breaks and the time the exercises are performed can be extended as necessary to alleviate symptoms. The 20-20-20 rule is further discussed at the end of this chapter in the Computer Vision Syndrome section. You may lengthen the number of seconds or frequency as needed.

The ciliary muscles can become "lazy" or weak in one eye when one eye is dominant. Lazy ciliary muscles or "lazy eye" can develop in a non dominant eye or when one eye has better visual acuity that the other.[12] Some people will turn their heads to the left or right while observing objects or walking to allow their dominant eye a greater field of vision. The ciliary muscle and lens in the dominate eye can also become overworked.

You can identify a possibly lazy eye with this simple test before you begin vision therapy. Cover either eye with your hand and focus at an object that may be somewhat blurry i.e. near the farthest range of your clear visual field. Do not close the eye that you are not focusing through, as this could make the vision in that closed eye blurry when it is opened. If you see the object better in one eye verses the other, or the object appears blurry in one eye, the difference in visual acuity could create an eye dominance issue that could lead to a "lazy" eye. If you feel strain in one eye more than your other eye while focusing up close, the eye experiencing the strain is likely to be your dominant eye. Eye dominance can create problems in the visual system when the dominate eye is being heavily relied on for the majority of visual perception.

If there is a difference in visual acuity between your two eyes, pick an object that you can see clearly with the dominant eye but that is blurry in the non dominant eye. Cover your dominant eye and with you weaker eye "manually" try to adjust your focus on the object by looking either in front of or behind the object. In order to accomplish this, you may have to close your eye or squint and then slowly open or unsquint as you concentrate on relaxing the eye in the process. While focusing on the object, try looking just beyond and also in front of the object. If the object becomes clearer while you do this, or after performing the eye exercises contained in this program, the visual difference in your eye most likely is the result of a calibration problem between your ciliary muscle, lens, and the correct focal point on the retina. If the object becomes clearer while squinting or looking in front of or beyond the object in this exercise, open or unsquint your eye while attempting to maintain the clear image. Repeat the process until you can do so or your ability to do so improves. When you repeat this process, it should be easier to retain the clearer image. If you have a dominate eye, focus on the weaker eye in vision therapy to improve its visual acuity. Doing this should relieve accumulated stress in the dominant eye as it is better able to share visual tasks more equally with the weaker eye as its visual acuity improves. As covered in the vision therapy section you can also perform patch therapy to help correct eye dominance.

A calibration problem can also affect your ability to adjust your focus in an eye whose shape has temporarily changed as a result of stress or aging. The ciliary muscle should automatically adjust the focal point to the proper spot on the retina. Vision therapy and the previous exercise will help to correct this condition.

How Corrective Lenses Harm Eyesight

It is commonly accepted that getting a set of eyeglasses or contact lenses is the right treatment for poor eyesight. When you consider the science, one can see that corrective lenses are actually worsening the condition of your eye. The results can be the same with Lasik or laser type surgeries that change the shape of the lens.

If once good vision has deteriorated, your visual system is likely placing your focal point at a spot that is either too far in front of or behind the proper location on the retina. This condition will result in a blurry image. This can be the same problem for those who have had poor visual acuity from birth or from a young age. Absent disease, a strained ciliary muscle and/or an inflexible lens may be at fault. Your focal point may be only slightly off the proper location on the retina at first. Over time though, the deviation can grow and larger deteriorations in visual acuity can occur. The decrease in the sharpness of the image may not be noticeable. The change can happen slowly; you may not be able to notice your vision deteriorating until you visit an optometrist or otherwise have your eyesight tested. To correct this condition an optometrist may simply prescribe corrective lenses. After an optometrist visit you most likely will be informed that you need a correction in the form of eyeglasses or contact lenses. If you get the correction, one of two things happen; one, your eyes will receive permanent relief from a temporary problem and adjust to the corrective lens where the same prescription strength is maintained, or two, your eyes will adjust to the corrective lens and your visual acuity will continue to deteriorate further. If the second situation results it will likely be determined at some point in the future that you need a stronger corrective prescription and your optometrist will prescribe you a stronger corrective lens. In either situation, you become less able to discard the lens correction; your eyes will either adjust to the lens and you will become stuck with it, or your vision will continue to deteriorate.

The addition of another lens to the visual system does not address the cause of the problem. The additional lens creates an adjustment in accommodation by changing the focal point in the eye. The added lens prevents the ciliary muscle from making the necessary adjustment of the focal point to achieve clear visual acuity. The ciliary muscle continues to hold the lens in an incorrect shape that places the focal point at an improper location on the retina; but the additional lens adjusts that location to the right place on the retina. The addition of another lens reinforces the wrong focal point as well as the incorrect shape of the lens that the ciliary muscle is maintaining.

Corrective lenses cannot properly increase your visual acuity. If you continue to engage in the same visual practices that caused the decrease in visual acuity, further deterioration in visual acuity is likely. When there is further deterioration in vision acuity the solutions are usually limited to stronger prescriptions. *Neither eyeglasses nor Lasik surgery improve accommodation, maintain lens elasticity, or strengthen or reduce accumulated stress in the ciliary muscle.*[13]

Dr. Bates and others continuing his research found that eyeglasses although initially helping vision and making reading more comfortable, act as a "crutch", and do not treat the underlying cause of the visual error.

Neither eyeglasses nor contact lenses can improve eyesight to the quality of uncorrected 20/20 vision. This concept can be very simply demonstrated by looking at any color in the color spectrum though a strong convex or concave glass. The color is always less intense when seen through the glass than when seen with the naked eye. Since the perception of form depends upon the perception of color, it follows that both color and form are not able to be seen as distinctly through eyeglasses or any lens for that matter. Even flat clear pane glass lowers the quality of vision in both color and form.

It is evident that eyeglasses do not improve visual acuity and may damage it further, as one cannot see clearly through them unless they produce and maintain the exact degree of refractive error they are designed to correct. This dependency cannot help improve visual acuity and should be expected to make the condition worse. As a matter of common experience, it does make the condition worse. Without some type of intervention, eyeglass prescriptions never decrease in strength they always increase in strength.

Research has shown that the refractive errors that may be present in an uncorrected eye have been found to never remain constant, they always change. As the refractive abnormalities have been found to continually change from day to day and even *hour to hour*, the accurate "fitting" of eyeglasses is impossible. To correct and improve visual acuity the accommodation abilities of the eye must be changed and improved.

Patients that are diagnosed with high degrees of myopia and hyperopia usually have great difficulty in becoming accustomed to full eyeglass correction. They often are never able to do so. Strong concave glasses for myopes make objects seem much smaller, while strong convex glasses enlarge them.

Optometrists, like other doctors, follow the medical model of correcting problems. They do as they are taught. Most believe that it is better to immediately fix a client's visual problems than refer them to possible months of visual therapy or stress reduction techniques. Your optometrist may purposely neglect to inform you about possible alternative solutions such as vision therapy that are likely to prove to be 100 percent successful. In doing so, either they or their colleagues are likely to gain a regular patient for as long as the patient lives. This ideology is changing with some eye care professionals, albeit a slow process. The fact that an eye care professional can get a board certification in vision therapy substantiates and gives further credibility to vision therapy. That vision therapy must be delivered in the professional's office though, subject to office visit and insurance charges, detracts from the credibility of some of these eye care professionals.

When people who wear eyeglasses go without them for a week or two, they frequently observe that their sight has improved. Sight always improves, to a greater or less degree, in the right conditions when glasses are discarded, although the improvement may not always be noted.

If you are a wearer of eyeglasses or contacts, try going without them for a week or two. If it is not feasible for you to remove your eyeglasses for whatever reasons, try to remove your eyeglasses and go without them to see as often as possible throughout your day. If this is not possible, try switching your eyeglasses and adjusting your vision to the next lower strength corrective lens prescription, or use the lower strength prescription as often as possible. When you are engaging in vision therapy, try to complete the exercises and activities without your corrective lenses.

What Makes an Effective Vision Therapy Program?

One may have many questions when evaluating a visual therapy program.

Are all vision therapy programs created equal?

Are optometrist and ophthalmologist administered programs different than self administered programs?

Are $1,800, $180, or $80 self administered vision therapy programs similar, or are they very different?

A vision therapy program is effective when adhering to it relieves accumulated stress in the eye, maintains lens flexibility, and strengthens the accommodation abilities of the eye resulting in increased visual acuity. A good vision therapy program will educate you and help you to identify and eliminate poor visual practices that can damage or reduce your visual acuity. An effective vision therapy program will help you identify and select the right eye exercises and visual activities for your specific eye deficiency, and help you determine how to perform them.

An effective vision therapy program should:

- Help you to identify and mitigate or eliminate visual practices that increase eye strain.
- Help you incorporate good visual practices and make them habitual
- Provide eye exercises and visual activities to increase your eye focusing power and accommodation based on your specific sight deficiencies.
- Help you determine which eye exercises to concentrate on to improve your specific sight deficiencies.

- Help you to identify what eye exercises and visual activities decrease eye strain based on your visual practices.

- Increase the focusing power of the eye for specific objects at varying distances

- Help you identify when to change or rotate through eye exercises based on your progress and your required risky visual practices such as working on a computer screen all day or reading for long periods of time.

A good vision therapy system will provide different therapy options for different visual deficiencies. You will find that certain vision therapy activities will relax your visual system; others will strengthen your ability to focus quickly, eliminate eye dominance issues, or will coordinate both of your eyes to work better together.

When you find the right vision therapy exercises that work for your condition, stick with them and be diligent about performing them. Be willing to change or vary those exercises as your visual practices improve. If you are mitigating the effects of necessary visual practices such as looking at a computer screen all day i.e. Computer Vision Syndrome, your needs will most likely stay consistent. Reevaluate and adjust your vision therapy program if necessary by rotating in different eye exercises, at intervals you determine. In performing vision therapy eye exercises and visual activities you will also learn more about how certain visual practices affect your visual acuity and how you can change or mitigate those visual practices to prevent eyestrain when they are required during your day.

A program's effectiveness is not based on its cost or how many bells, whistles, lights, and/or special equipment that it has. If a program addresses these listed items, the results that you see from the program will most likely be from your persistence in following the program verses any special equipment, lights, eye charts, or cost of the vision therapy program you follow.

What is Computer Vision Syndrome?

The American Optometric Association (http://www.aoa.org) describes Computer Vision Syndrome or CVS as the visual symptoms or deficiencies that arise from looking at a computer screen. Many of these symptoms can be broadly classified as asthenopia, an ophthalmological term for eyestrain. Most of the symptoms are associated with other forms of near work. Symptoms include; eyestrain (non-specific ocular discomfort), blurred distant vision, blurred near vision, diplopia (double vision), fatigue, dry or irritated eyes, headache, and neck and/or backaches.[14]

Those who specialize in vision therapy agree that people who spend more than two hours a day on the computer are likely to be affected by Computer Vision Syndrome. The American Optometric Association reports that as many as 50 to 90 percent of people who work on computer screens and display terminals regularly develop visual problems as a result. Reading for prolonged periods at close fixed distances can cause the same symptoms.

The extent that an individual experiences visual symptoms from Computer Vision Syndrome often depends on their current level of visual acuity and the amount of time they spend looking at a computer screen. Visual acuity problems such as nearsightedness, farsightedness, astigmatism, eye dominance, etc., can contribute to the development of Computer Vision Syndrome symptoms.

If acute, the CVS symptoms are only temporary and will dissipate soon after the cessation of computer work. In chronic cases, some people may continue to experience visual symptoms such as blurred vision at distances even after cessation of the activities that caused CVS. If the visual activities continue and no action is taken to address CVS, symptoms are likely to recur and increase in severity and longevity. In time, these symptoms usually worsen and can reoccur without engaging in the activity that originally caused CVS.

There are some visual practices that can be changed to reduce the symptoms experienced from CVS. Taking steps to control lighting and glare on the computer screen, establishing proper working distances, and maintaining correct body posture for computer viewing to reduce muscle stress, are ways to help minimize the symptoms of CVS.

Another practice that those with symptoms of Computer Vision Syndrome can perform is to blink more frequently. Those who work on computers for extended periods have been found to blink about five times less than average. Blinking less frequently causes tears to evaporate more quickly and leads to less eye moisture or dryer eyes. Those who blink slowly 10 times every 20 minutes re-moisturize their eyes. As many tissues in the eye like the cornea receive oxygen and nutrients from tears, this can help to prevent irritation and provide the necessary nutrients to maintain healthy tissue regeneration.

Most importantly, Computer Vision Syndrome symptoms most often occur when one looks at a computer screen for too long of a period of time without taking appropriate breaks. Using the 20-20-20 rule helps prevent eyestrain. The 20-20-20 rule calls for one to look away from the screen at an object that is at least 20 feet away, every 20 minutes, for 20 seconds. Another way to relieve accumulated stress from building up in the eye is to look away from the computer screen at an object that is far away from you for 10 to 15 seconds (over 100 meters) and then look at an closer object closer to you (20 meters) for 10 to 15 seconds and performing this sequence 10 times every 20 minutes. If eye dominance is also present, it would be helpful to perform this activity for each eye independently while the other eye is covered and not closed.

Relieving accumulated eye strain by performing vision therapy at the appropriate break intervals is another option that is very effective for both treatment and prevention of CVS.

Pinhole Glasses

Pinhole glasses typically are plastic glasses with non transparent lenses that have many tiny holes. Pinhole glasses usually have about 180 to 250 1mm diameter holes straight through each eyeglass lens. These holes serve to reduce the width and variance of the many diverging light rays that are reflected off of the different shapes and objects in your line of sight. Any lens will not focus all light rays perfectly; a "point" of focus on the retina is normally imaged as a spot rather than a precise point. The size of the spot that a lens produces is often referred to as the circle of confusion; the more precise that circle is, the better the resulting visual acuity. Blurred vision can also be due to the spot being focused either in front of the retina in the case of nearsightedness, or behind the retina in farsightedness. Each hole in the lenses of pinhole glasses restricts divergent light rays and only allows much narrower beams of light to enter the eye from the object you are focusing on. Without the divergent light waves, the lens is better able to focus the narrow beams of light that reach it and pass through it after bring reflected off of the object in view. The narrower light beams are better focused, resulting in a reduction in the size of the circle of confusion on the retina which increases the sharpness of the image.

Looking through the pinholes of the lenses can be somewhat difficult because the field of vision is blocked by the plastic of the lenses that the pinholes are placed in. You must find a hole or holes to look through to view an object. The resulting vision is much clearer. Objects that previously were not in focus can often be seen clearly.

When wearing pinhole glasses the immediate improvement in visual acuity can be amazing. This concept is well understood by optometrists and ophthalmologists. Pinhole glasses are often used in eye testing to determine the best correctable vision that a person has. If a person is not able to read the 20/20 eye test line even with correction, the test is done through pinholes. If the person still cannot see to 20/20, it could indicate the presence of further abnormalities or eye disease, and further examination would be required.

It is claimed that wearing pinhole glasses will re-train the eyes to focus correctly. There are a number of thoughts as to how this happens; one is that the pinhole glasses relax the ciliary muscles; another is that it recalibrates the way the brain works with the visual system.

If experimenting with or using pinhole glasses, it is recommended that they be worn outside or in places of bright illumination. The holes of these plastic glasses only allow beams of light in specific trajectories into the eye; they also prevent other beams of light from reaching the eye. This reduces the amount of light that reaches the lens and retina, which can result in poorer quality vision in dim or low light situations. When these glasses are worn for any period of time, you may "feel your eye working" or your eyes may "get tired." The benefit of this is unclear. Some package inserts or instructions attached to pinhole glasses claim that total permanent correction of visual acuity is possible. Under a legal settlement with the Federal Trade Commission, the companies that manufacture or sell these glasses can no longer make these claims in the United States.

Some people claim they experience visual acuity improvement with these glasses while others claim they have received no benefit. While the benefit may be unclear, wearing these glasses will not harm your eyes.

If you choose to wear or experiment with pinhole glasses, any activities you engage in should not include anything that requires depth perception or anything else that is dangerous or where your safety could be at risk. You should not drive or operate machinery.

If there is an improvement in your eyesight with pinhole glasses, there is an excellent chance that improvement can become permanent and also that vision therapy will improve your visual acuity.

Chapter 5 Additional Factors to Consider

Protecting Your Eyesight

There are many factors that can determine how well vision therapy programs work. Generally speaking, it is important to understand that most of the factors that determine how effective a vision therapy program can be are the same factors that influence and determine good physical and mental health.

What additional factors should be considered to naturally improve eyesight?

Some of the most imperative factors are:

- Whether a general disease or eye disease is present, and if so, understanding any limitations that the disease presents.
- Understanding the effects of any medications that you are taking
- Controlling the effects of aging
- Proper diet and nutrition, including toxic chemicals in processed food that you may unknowingly be ingesting
- Controlling physical and mental stress

It is never too late to implement measures to protect your vision or your overall health.

Disease

A decline in visual acuity can occur from many things besides eye strain, the calibration of the ciliary muscle or inflexibility of the lens. There are many general diseases of the body that can increase your risk of eye disease.

Vision therapy is not meant to treat eye disease or take the place of an eye or medical doctor in the treatment of disease. Although most diseases can be controlled or prevented by proper diet and nutrition, exercise, and controlling stress, if you have an eye related or vision problem, or other medical problem, you should see a doctor for general diagnosis and medical treatment options.

It is important that you rule out eye disease or other general diseases of the body as causes for deteriorating vision. The following diseases or conditions can all contribute to and reduce visual acuity:

1. Diabetes

2. High blood pressure

3. Heart disease - cardiovascular disorders impair circulation to the eyes

4. Smoking - depletes antioxidants i.e. addiction

5. Poor diet and nutrition

6. Vitamin deficiency

7. Some prescription drugs - certain prescription drugs can reduce or deteriorate visual acuity.

It is important for good visual acuity and overall physical health to receive regular or annual physicals, health risk assessments, and/or diagnosis and care for disease. Talk to your doctor to eliminate disease as a possible cause or contributing factor of deteriorating visual acuity and/or to receive medical treatment for a diagnosed disease.

As good as a resource as your doctor can be; *do not rely only on your doctor as a sole source for information. Do your own research regarding your particular situation or ailment.* There are many medical books, publications, studies, and other relevant information sources that are made available to the general public for research through direct sale, public libraries, colleges, and the internet. If using the internet as a source, at a minimum be sure to triple check the information you find as well as perform additional research on the *sources* of the information.

Many general diseases of the body as well as eye disease can be symptoms of the same root problem that can be effectively treated with proper diet and nutrition, physical exercise, and controlling stress.

Medication

Pharmaceutical medications that "treat" chronic or acute disease or illness can have profound side effects on the body and on visual acuity. Prior to ingesting any drug, you must understand all of a particular drug's potential side effects as well as the potential interactions of all medications you ingest. Your doctor or pharmacist may not discuss a drug's side effects with you in detail or may only mention the most common side effects.

Be sure to thoroughly read the medication package insert and as well as any related medical studies to understand the side effects of medication you take. The Physician's Desk Reference (PDR) is another resource of information for your prescription drug. The PDR can be found online at www.pdr.net.

You can also get drug information from the U.S. Food and Drug Administration at www.fda.gov.

Drug clinical trial testing results for specific drugs is made available online at www.clinicaltrials.gov, and through medical journals available at www.pubmed.gov.

Aging

You will age, but how you age is critical and is something that is within your ability to control. Proper diet and nutrition, vitamin and mineral supplementation, physical exercise, stress control, and avoiding smoking or being exposed to smoke, are important ways to help control the negative effects of aging and reduce your chances of eye problems. Addressing these items will ease the effects of aging and help mitigate the emergence of disease. In the healthy environment that is created by good habits, vision therapy is even more effective in improving visual acuity.

With the increased dependence on medications, the reduced nutritional content in foods, the chemical additives found in all processed food, the increase in obesity, disease, stress, and tension, and the amount of time spent on cell phones and in front of computer screens and television, it is no wonder 90 percent of people will need glasses to correct developed visual deficiencies and blurred vision.

The effects of aging can be controlled by diet and nutrition, exercise, and stress relief.

Diet and Nutrition

Maintaining proper diet and nutrition is probably the single best way to protect your eyesight. Consuming the correct foods in the right combinations, amounts, and at the right times are all important for your body to function properly.

The type of food that you eat is essential to your health. More food is available for consumption today than ever before.

Unfortunately, much of this food is not good for you; it either contains too much of the wrong nutrients (sugar, chemicals, unhealthy fat), or too little of the right nutrients (vitamins, minerals, protein, essential fatty acids). Many popular and mouth-watering foods do not have any nutritional value at all. Nearly every person could and should significantly reduce the amount of calories they get from simple carbohydrates, chemical preservatives, additives, and/or sweeteners.

Generally speaking, there are foods that are nutritious and that provide good building blocks and fuel for your body, and foods that you should not eat because they contain chemicals or ingredients that poison and are destructive to your body. For the most part, absent a food sensitivity or food allergy, you cannot go wrong abiding by the four basic food groups (meat and egg, whole grain, vegetable and fruit, and dairy groups). Choose naturally raised animal products that are grass fed, free range, or that have natural diets. Choose fruits and vegetables that are organic and grown in soils that have not been depleted of minerals.

Sugar and Sweeteners

Among the most dangerous food ingredients are sugar and sugar related sweeteners such as high fructose corn syrup.

Eating causes your blood sugar to go up. How much and how fast it rises depends on the type of food you ate, the amount of the food, the combinations of different foods eaten, and your body.

Your body releases the hormone insulin in response to increases in blood sugar. Insulin takes sugar out of your blood and puts it into your cells. In the majority of sedentary people who eat a lot of carbohydrates, especially simple carbohydrates such as sugar or other sweeteners, blood sugar levels rise and remain elevated. To manage the high blood sugar levels, the body must release higher amounts of insulin to take sugar out of the bloodstream and lower the blood sugar level. Over time, as a result of high insulin levels, the cells of the body become more and more resistant to the effects of insulin. This is called insulin resistance, which results in the body releasing even more insulin to control blood sugar. In sedentary or non active people, insulin cannot place all or most of the sugar from the blood stream into the muscle cells to be stored and burnt as energy in muscle cell activity. In sedentary people, the mitochondria in the muscle cell cannot store as much sugar for energy as active people. If the muscle cells are not actively burning energy and cannot store any more energy, the body has only one place for the sugar to go. The insulin causes the sugar to be placed into fat cells that convert the sugar into adipose tissue or fat, the body's way of storing caloric energy. Your body becomes better and better at storing any excess sugar calories as fat. The result is that a person eating high simple carbohydrate diets are likely to experience high blood sugar levels that result in low blood sugar levels once high circulating insulin levels act. Blood sugar roller coasters can cause large scale mood swings and cravings, and make it very difficult for people to lose undesirable fat body weight. The body will also not burn fat while it has high circulating levels of sugar and insulin.

When you eat or drink a food item that contains a high quantity of simple sugars, your blood sugar level can rise very quickly. This causes the pancreas to release a large amount of insulin, which in turn removes too much sugar from the blood. The result is that you end up with a blood sugar level that is too low. This causes you to feel both tired and irritable. Your blood sugar level will eventually normalize, but this reoccurring process is very damaging to your body. Studies have shown that rapid fluctuations in the blood sugar level can cause bizarre reactions in individuals comparable to behaviors of those with mental disease.

Besides radical behavior and mood changes, excessive sugar consumption is linked to Type 2 diabetes. Diabetes is among the highest contributors to death in the world. Diabetes does not usually kill you directly; it opens the door for other diseases to emerge by lowering your immune system, or interfering with the amounts of hormones that your body produces. On hot and humid days, consuming large amounts of sugar is more harmful to your body than ingesting poison. In these situations, sugar also interferes with the way that your body uses water to keep itself cool.

Diabetes leads to obesity. Obesity creates conditions in the body that are optimal for disease. Obesity is also among the highest contributors to death in the world. For those that are overweight, constant sugar consumption such as drinking soda pop, gives your body a steady supply of simple carbohydrate energy. This sugar energy is glucose that immediately goes into your blood stream and must be used as energy by the body, placed in cell mitochondria, or converted to energy storage as fat. It is the first source of energy that the body uses for fuel. The combination of calories from sugar as well as any food that you may have eaten can leave the body with many extra calories. When the body has a constant steady supply of excess calories from high sugar foods such as soda pop, it has no alternative but to store the extra calories as body fat.

To prevent this from happening, eliminate sugary foods and drinks or at a minimum, abstain from snacking on them between meals. Avoid everything that contains significant amounts of processed simple sugars such as soda pop and candy, sweetened cereals, or anything else that is artificially sweetened, or that contains a high amount or percentage of sugar calories in comparison to overall calories. This is especially true of most bottled beverages.

To repeat, eliminate eating sugary foods and drinks or at least at a minimum, abstain from snacking on them between meals.

Fat

Foods that are fried, or cooked in saturated or non saturated fats represent another risk. Most fats increase the total amount of calories in food and your risk of obesity and heart disease.

Stay away from all foods or snacks that are cooked or fried, in fat or oil. Even small amounts of foods that contain high amounts of fat or sugar will always have more empty calories than nutritional value.

Foods that are higher in fat will not produce satiety as quickly as lower fat foods. Satiety is the feeling of fullness that helps you to know when to stop eating. Fatty foods are calorie dense which increases the probability you will over eat.

Hydrogenated oils present an additional risk. These oils are prevalent in many foods such as non natural peanut butter that does not require refrigeration after opening. Hydrogenated oils are found in nearly all cooking oils therefore they are present in nearly all foods that are fried. These oils can interfere with the body's normal processes of utilizing eicosanoids to activate hormones. Eicosanoids are hormonal signaling molecules derived from essential fatty acids and are used by the body to immediately activate inactive hormones found floating in the blood. Eicosanoids and essential fatty acids are essential components in the process of activating and utilizing hormones that are freely circulating in the blood waiting to be put to use.

Processed Packaged Foods

As a general rule, anything processed and contained in a package is not healthy for you to eat. Processed packaged food items usually contain chemical additives, preservatives, or genetically modified organisms. The exceptions to unsafe packaged foods are non processed foods where the packaging simply holds natural food together such as bags of nuts, fruits and vegetables or butchered meats. Dehydrated or freeze dried foods may also be safe to eat if they do not contain chemicals and preservatives.

Do not eat processed meats. Choose the meat of animals raised in natural environments and on their natural diets. Animals that have been raised in close quarters with other animals that have been fattened up on genetically modified corn and kept healthy by injections of antibiotics are not as healthy for you as free range animals that have been raised on natural grass fed diets. As these meats are more expensive, find a good affordable local meat supplier. Less quantity of a higher quality meat is better for your body.

Those with diets of only fresh fruits and vegetables and high quality free range animal meats will create a healthy environment that is resistant to the effects of aging.

Food Allergies

If you have a food sensitivity or food allergy you should be careful to eliminate those foods from your diet.

If you have a disease or ailment, even if it seems unrelated to your diet such as nervous system or autoimmune diseases, you should receive a high quality test for food allergies. Many ailments that appear to be "diseases" can actually be a food allergy. Food allergies can cause severe autoimmune disorders that are extremely difficult to diagnose.

Again, chose naturally raised animal products that are grass fed, free range, or that have natural diets. Choose fruits and vegetables that are organic and grown in soils that have not been depleted of minerals. Prepare healthy snacks such as fruits or nuts if you get hungry between meals.

Genetically Modified Foods

GMOs ("genetically modified organisms") are living organisms whose genetic material (DNA) has been artificially manipulated in a laboratory through genetic engineering. This relatively new science creates unstable combinations of plant, animal, bacterial and/or viral genes that do not occur naturally in nature or that are possible through traditional crossbreeding methods.[15] It allows selected genes to be transferred from one organism into another, even between nonrelated species.

Many developed nations do not consider GMOs to be safe. In more than 60 countries around the world, including Australia, Japan, and all of the countries in the European Union, there are significant restrictions or outright bans on the production and sale of GMOs. In the U.S., the government has approved GMOs based on studies conducted by the same corporations that created the GMOs and profit from their sale.

Unfortunately, even though polls in the U.S. consistently show that a significant majority of Americans want to know if the food they are purchasing contains GMOs, the powerful biotech lobby has succeeded in keeping this information from the public.[16]

GMO plants are genetically engineered to either be resistant to certain types of pesticide or to produce their own pesticide internally. The health effects of GMOs are mired in controversy. A study performed in 2012 made headlines around the world with its shocking photos of rats that developed large tumors after eating Monsanto's genetically modified maize, whether or not it was treated with Monsanto's Roundup weed killer. The publisher retracted the study, but it was clear that the publisher was forced to do this based on pressure from "economic interests."[17]

GMOs that produce their own pesticide internally kill insects by dissolving their digestive tracks. Although GMO seed producers state that GMOs do not have the same effect in people, GMOs stand accused of creating digestive problems, which can then lead to food allergies and autoimmune disorders.

GMO's can be found in many food items including vitamins. As nearly all of commercially produced corn and soy in the United States is from GMO seed, GMOs are in nearly every processed and packaged food item. To avoid GMOs one needs to avoid eating anything with a corn or soy byproduct. The following is a partial list of these byproducts showing their prevalence. According to the FDA, food products containing these ingredients cannot be labeled as "natural."

- Calcium carbonate - calcium supplement containing starch made from GMO corn
- Corn syrup - food syrup made from GMO corn
- Dextrose monohydrate - corn syrup based sweetener containing starch made from GMO corn
- Glycerin – food additive used for taste and to retain moisture in foods that is sometimes made from GMO rapeseed (canola oil)
- High fructose corn syrup - industrial food product sweetener made from GMO corn
- Maltodextrin - food thickening additive usually made from GMO corn starch
- Sodium bicarbonate - baking soda containing GMO ingredients used for things such as making dough rise
- Soy lecithin - an ingredient made from GMO soy that is included in many packaged foods
- Soy protein isolate - a dry powder food ingredient made from GM soybean plants

- Tocopherols - an ingredient derived from or contained in some vitamin E that is commonly made from GM soy, corn or cotton

It is highly recommended that you avoid all GMOs and GMO byproducts, including meat from animals raised on GMOs.

For more information about how to avoid GMO products, visit the "NON GMO Project" at http://www.nongmoproject.org.

Chemical Sweeteners and Preservatives

Aspartame is used as a substitute sweetener in thousands of products as 'alternative' to sugar. Most diet sodas, low calorie sweetened drinks, and candies, as well as many processed foods contain it.

Aspartame may not be marketed by its real name, but through brands such as Equal and NutraSweet. The marketing strategy of using different brands to sell into the consumer market may be due to the fact that aspartame has been identified as a known and extremely dangerous Excitotoxin. An excitotoxin 'excites' cells in the body into overproducing certain particular chemicals that cause them to malfunction or burn out prematurely. Aspartame particularly affects nerve cells.

To determine if a food item contains aspartame check the ingredients on the package. Aspartame should be listed as an ingredient on the product package.

The harmful effects of consuming an aspartame sweetened product can manifest themselves through a number of neurological problems and symptoms like headaches, fatigue, vision problems, and anxiety. Ongoing consumption of this excitotoxin can cause symptoms to progress and possibly worsen, until the toxin is eliminated from the diet completely.

Aspartame is considered physically addictive, a chemical dependency begins to form when aspartame is consumed regularly and this addiction can be very hard to break. The chemical dependency developed through consumption creates an ongoing demand for products that contain aspartame. This is evidenced by the many people who cannot seem to quit drinking diet soft drinks containing aspartame, even after they are made aware of the extremely dangerous risks and experience serious related health problems.

Due to the neurological effects of aspartame, its continued use can be expected to lead to many forms of neurological diseases including cancer. Aspartame has been suggested as a prominent cause for certain forms of brain cancer.

One study actually found that 67 percent of female rats exposed to aspartame developed tumors roughly the size of golf balls or larger.[18]

Aspartame is created using Monsanto's genetically modified bacteria.[19] Aspartame is a byproduct, derived from the fecal waste of the bacteria.

It is highly recommended that you avoid this addictive drug-like substance at any cost, and replace it with a healthy alternative such as honey or stevia.

Monosodium Glutamate (MSG) is also an excitotoxin. As an excitotoxin, the harmful effects of MSG can be similar to that of aspartame. It is a flavor enhancer used to make food taste much better and enhance its desirability. MSG is considered to be physically addictive, which increases the demand for products that contain it. MSG can be called a number of different names in a list of ingredients.[20]

Glutamic Acid	Anything "hydrolyzed"	Soy Protein Concentrate
Glutamate		
Monosodium Glutamate	Any "hydrolyzed protein"	Soy Protein Isolate
Monopotassium Glutamate	Calcium Caseinate	Whey Protein
Calcium Glutamate	Sodium Caseinate	Whey Protein Concentrate
Monoammonium Glutamate	Yeast Food	Whey Protein Isolate
Magnesium Glutamate	Yeast Nutrient	Anything "...protein"
	Autolyzed Yeast	
Natrium Glutamate	Gelatin	Vetsin
	Textured Protein	Ajinomoto
Yeast Extract	Soy Protein	Natural Flavors

Depending on how a food is made, the FDA might not require a manufacturer to list MSG on the label. The majority of packaged foods contain MSG or similar and related ingredients. It is recommended that you stay away from all packaged and manufactured foods.

Excitotoxins cause excitotoxicity, which not only destroys the nervous system but causes obesity. It is theorized that excitoxins increase one's desire to consume carbohydrates and sugars over protein rich foods which is a major contributor to obesity.[21]

How to Eat

How you eat is important. Many people eat only one meal at one time per day. They may eat nothing else for the rest of the day or eat unhealthy snacks. Whether this practice is intentional in order to reduce calories for losing weight or not, this practice of eating is counterproductive.

Countless studies and experiments have shown that how you eat plays a vital role in how your body utilizes and stores fat. In some of these experiments, people were put on restricted diets, or provided fewer calories than their bodies burned daily. One group was provided their total amount of restricted calories in many small meals spread throughout the day. The second group was provided the same amount of restricted calories, but they were required to eat all of the calories in only one meal per day. Because both groups were eating fewer calories than they burned daily, both groups lost weight. The significant differences in the two groups did not become apparent until the participants in the studies returned to their normal dietary habits. Upon resuming normal eating habits, the group that ate all of their calories in one large meal gained more weight in fat than the group that ate their calories in small meals. During the period of restricted calorie intake, the bodies of those who ate the large meals once per day, adapted to the stress of "famine" (reduced calories in one meal) by slowing down their basal metabolic rate (energy required to maintain normal body functions) and gearing the body towards storing any available excess calories to be better prepared for any similar calorie deprivation situations in the future. When these individuals returned to normal eating patterns, their bodies more readily stored all of the excess calories in their diet as fat to stockpile energy for future periods of starvation.

Even though the experiment was performed initially with restricted calories, the harmful effects of eating large meals once per day also applies to those who are not dieting or restricting their caloric intake, as the body can only store so much glucose as glycogen in the muscles and liver to be used as energy throughout the day. This stored glycogen energy varies from individual to individual but it will not supply the body for long, therefore the remaining excess calories from one large meal must be stored as fat as the body has no other way to store these excess calories.

It is recommended that food be eaten in 3-5 meals spread throughout equally throughout the day 3-4 hours apart depending on how much you sleep, especially if you are dieting or eating restricted calories. When you eat in smaller more frequent meals, you provide your body with a constant supply of steady calories that it needs to burn throughout the day. Eating in this way helps the body to understand that it will receive a steady supply of calories and prevent it from adapting to potential periods of starvation by slowing the metabolism and gearing up to store excess calories as fat whenever they are available.

Do not eat before going to bed at night. You last meal should be 3-4 hours before you go to bed or any excess calories that are digested during this period of sleep inactivity are likely to be stored as fat.

Eating before you go to bed can also make your body work harder to digest the food you have eaten and keep you from getting a good night's sleep. Digestion at night can also impact essential hormones from cycling properly.

Both the quality and quantity of your sleep are important factors in controlling stress.

Vitamin and Mineral Supplements

The government calculates a recommended daily allowance (RDA) of vitamins and minerals for you. The RDA is determined by calculating the lowest amount of each vitamin and mineral that you can take without falling into a diseased state due to a nutritional deficiency. This means that if you only receive the maximum RDA of vitamins and minerals for your recommended group on a daily basis, you are on the brink of falling into a diseased state because you are not getting enough vitamins or minerals for your body to function at full capacity. If you are physically active and fall into the higher need percentile for your age group, the RDA will not be enough to meet your nutritional needs. If you are placing higher demands on your body your requirements for vitamins and minerals increase, therefore if you are getting only the RDA, you are likely to be in or close to a diseased state. Your body needs more than the RDA of vitamins and minerals to be able to complete normal bodily functions efficiently.

Women should be sure that they are getting enough iron in their diet as they are at risk of becoming deficient in iron due to their menstrual period. This can also lead to the development of diseases such as osteoporosis.

A vitamin or mineral deficiency can result in a number of symptoms, including the inability to produce essential hormones, lowering of the immune system, or the feeling that you have no energy or motivation. Vitamin deficiencies will cause you to age prematurely affecting the way you look and feel.

Studies have shown that low levels of antioxidant vitamins (vitamin E, C, and various carotenoids), increase your risk of cataracts, macular degeneration and other diseases of the eye.

Nutritional supplementation of high quality vitamins and minerals is the best way to ensure you will meet your nutritional requirements. As most fruit and vegetables are grown in mineral depleted soils and animals are fed GMO grain from mineral depleted soils, the added supplementation of enough of the right vitamins and minerals to meet the needs of the body is an absolute necessity. Supplementing with enough of the right vitamins and minerals will ensure that your body is able to maintain normal functions including proper hormonal ratios, cycles, and balances to combat the effects of aging.

A vitamin and mineral supplement is highly recommended; research vitamin and mineral products to determine which one is right for you. If you are not knowledgeable in these areas or prefer to be advised, it is recommended that you seek the counsel of a holistic doctor to advise you on your vitamin and mineral needs, product identification, evaluation, and supplementation options.

Be smart and play it safe by supplementing your diet with a good form of vitamins and minerals.

Summary

Eliminating foods that contain high amounts of sugar, high fructose corn syrup, corn and/or soy oils, hydrogenated oils, GMO's, artificial additives and sweeteners, and supplementing with high quality vitamins and minerals is critical to anti-aging.

Additional Diet and Nutrition Resources for Overall Health

The importance of diet and nutrition on aging, overall health, and to maintain or improve the quality of your eyesight has been greatly emphasized in this book and cannot be overstated.

It is highly recommended that you take the time to learn more about how diet and nutrition affect aging and hormones and what you can do to limit or even reverse the effects of aging on your body and visual acuity.

Research has shown that some specific diets have enormous health benefits. Many people who have followed diets that advocate eating more protein while severely restricting carbohydrates have reported substantial reductions in body fat.

There has been a significant amount of attention given to many of the best selling diet books in this category; The Zone, Protein Power, Lean Bodies, The 5-Day Miracle Diet, Dr. Atkins New Diet Revolution, Paleo diet, and The Carbohydrate Addict's Diet.

Researchers have found that the fat you eat is not necessarily the fat you gain. The benefits are not limited to fat loss. It has been documented that some of the individuals who have gone on these diets have not only lost weight but lowered cholesterol and blood pressure, and reversed the onset of diseases, including heart disease, gout, and diabetes.

Any of the above listed books are recommended.

The following books are highly recommended:

- "The Anti-Aging Zone" by Dr. Barry Sears

- "Toxic Fat: When Good Fat Turns Bad" Dr. by Barry Sears.

Dr. Barry Sears is one of the world's most leading experts in the field of diet and nutrition and he has produced many books on these subjects. It is strongly suggested that you learn more about his philosophy to combat the effects of aging and it is strongly encouraged that you consider putting his methods into practice. There is no relationship monetarily or otherwise between this Author and Dr. Barry Sears.

"The Anti-Aging Zone" by Barry Sears

"Toxic Fat: When Good Fat Turns Bad" by Barry Sears

Dr. Barry Sears website: www.drsears.com

Physical Exercise

The benefits of physical exercise are numerous.

Physical exercise burns fat, boosts energy, improves muscle strength and endurance, delivers oxygen and nutrients to your tissues, and the helps the cardiovascular system to work more efficiently. Exercise helps prevent weight gain and prevents the Basal Metabolic Rate from adjusting lower in order to maintain weight loss during periods of caloric deprivation. Exercise boosts "good" cholesterol (HDL, high density lipoprotein) and decreases "bad" cholesterol (LDL, low density lipoprotein). Physical exercise is important in maintain proper healthy body functions like hormonal regulation and production, including growth hormone and testosterone or estrogen production. Physical exercise increases the quality of life and improves sex drive. Physical exercise reduces potential injuries, especially in osteoporosis and hip fractures, and promotes healing with common problems such as back pain. Exercise helps us to fall asleep quicker and to sleep more restfully.

Physical exercise helps to prevent depression and anxiety. Improved self esteem is one of the top benefits of regular physical activity. Exercising stimulates brain chemicals. Exercise causes your body to release chemicals called endorphins that can improve your mood and the way you feel about yourself. The feeling that follows physical exercise is often described as "euphoric" and is accompanied by an energizing outlook.

Physical exercise enhances cognitive function. Ample evidence exists, and many studies such as "The Caerphilly Heart Disease

Study" support, that exercise reduces the risk of developing dementia.

Physical exercise reduces stress. Physical exercise improves your mood, especially after stressful events and work days. Frequent and regular physical exercise boosts the immune system and helps to prevent diseases like heart disease, stroke, cardiovascular disease, Type 2 diabetes, cancer and obesity.

According to the World Health Organization, physical inactivity is the fourth leading risk factor for global mortality. The amount of physical activity is decreasing worldwide. Globally, 1 in 3 adults is not active enough.[22]

This section on physical exercise is not designed to be a complete guide as innumerable books and enormous amounts of information on the subject have been written and are readily available. It is meant to provide an overview and to emphasize the importance of exercise in creating the proper environment in your body to promote health, combat disease, and improve visual acuity.

Physical exercises are generally grouped into three types, depending on the overall effect they have on the human body:

- Stretching is referred to as flexibility training and is meant to lengthen your muscles. These exercises are meant to improve range of motion, increase joint flexibility and keep muscles limber, which helps to reduce the probability of injury.

- Aerobic exercise is any physical activity that puts large muscle groups to work causing your body to use more oxygen than it would while resting. The goal of aerobic exercise is to increase cardiovascular endurance and strengthen the heart. Some examples of aerobic exercise are; brisk walking, jogging, bicycling, rowing, and hiking.

- Anaerobic exercise is referred to as resistance or strength training, and can firm, strengthen, and tone your muscles, as well as improve coordination, balance, and bone strength. These exercises can be done with weights or body weight. There are many different types of anaerobic exercise, some examples are; weight training, bench press, squats, pushups, lunges, sprinting, and bicep curls with weight.

Although one should strive for doing all three types of physical exercise, any exercise from any group is better than doing nothing at all.

The World Health Organization makes recommendations on the amounts of physical activity for three (3) different age groups; 5–17 years old; 18–64 years old; and 65 years old and above.[23]

For adults aged 18 - 64 years, physical activity includes; leisure time physical activities (walking, dancing, gardening, hiking, swimming), transportation (walking, cycling), occupational (work), household chores, play, games, sports or planned exercise, in the context of daily, family, and community activities.

For adults aged 18–64 to improve cardio respiratory and muscular fitness, bone health, reduce the risk of NCDs and depression, it is recommended:

- At least 150 minutes of moderate-intensity aerobic physical activity throughout the week or do at least 75 minutes of vigorous-intensity aerobic physical activity throughout the week or an equivalent combination of moderate- and vigorous-intensity activity.

- Aerobic activity should be performed in bouts of at least 10 minutes duration.

- For additional health benefits, adults should increase their moderate-intensity aerobic physical activity to 300 minutes per week, or engage in 150 minutes of vigorous-intensity aerobic physical activity per week, or an equivalent combination of moderate- and vigorous-intensity activity.

- Muscle-strengthening activities should be done involving major muscle groups on two (2) or more days a week.

For further information go to www.who.int and download the complete World Health Organization document by searching for "Global Recommendations on Physical Activity for Health."

You do not need to set aside large chunks of time to exercise. You can do many little things to implement exercise into your daily schedule. Remember, any amount of exercise at any age is beneficial.

Here are some easy ways to work physical activity into your life:

- Minimize the use of your car and walk to destinations within a mile

- Stand instead of sit, while working, at meetings, or whenever you can

- Speed walk or walk briskly whenever you can

- Walk a couple blocks at lunch time, make an agreement with a friend to join you

- Take stairs instead of using the elevator, especially if you are only going a few floors

- Do 20 pushups, air squats, sit ups, or toe touches every hour, two hours, or at lunch

- Borrow a dog and take it for a walk every day

- Play with children, either your own or someone else's

- Turn on some music and dance
- Go to the park and play catch
- Bounce a small ball against the wall
- Flex different muscle groups while you are waiting in line
- Walk around the airport during layovers
- Park at the back of the lot when shopping or at work
- Get a pedometer and try to increase your steps daily
- Mow the lawn with a push mower
- Turn off the television
- Make a set time for a stretch break at work

Consider these exercise tips:

- Do an activity or something that you like
- Make a schedule and stick to it
- Workout at a time when you have the most energy
- Be efficient when you go to exercise
- Make a competition out of it or include a partner
- Keep your exercise session short if necessary, do something instead of nothing even if it is for five (5) minutes
- Reward yourself for achieving your exercise goals
- Make exercise fun and part of your lifestyle instead of something you "need" to do

As the interests of people can differ greatly, find a type of exercise, activity, or sport you think you might like do you and learn more about it. Hang out and spend time at places where people do the activity, and go try it out!

Be sure to get medical clearance before beginning any physical exercise program.

Stress Relief through Meditation and Relaxation

The importance of stress reduction on aging, overall health, proper functioning of the visual system, and the quality of your visual acuity has been greatly emphasized in this book.

In addition to physical exercise, is highly recommended that you engage in some form of general stress relief or employ some type of relaxation method such as meditation to control physical and mental stress and to prevent elevated levels of cortisol.

High levels of stress can have a number of negative effects on your body. High stress levels increase the production of cortisol and decrease testosterone levels in men.[24] Cortisol is the body's stress hormone. At sustained elevated levels, cortisol causes premature aging, slows down healing and normal cell regeneration, destroys healthy muscle and bone, weakens the immune system, and interferes with normal healthy endocrine function.

The problems associated with chronically elevated cortisol levels include:[25]

- Suppressed immunity
- Hypertension
- High blood sugar (hyperglycemia)
- Insulin resistance
- Carbohydrate cravings
- Metabolic syndrome and Type 2 diabetes
- Fat deposits on the face, neck, and belly

- Reduced libido
- Bone loss

Controlling overall stress can be a difficult and constant struggle for many people. High levels of stress are uncomfortable and can reduce the quality of sleep that is essential for the rejuvenation of the mind and body as well as the normal cycling of hormones and proper operation of the endocrine system.

Effective stress reduction methods may vary significantly from person to person. Each person may have drastically different methods to control or reduce stress. Methods may vary from spending time with loved ones to watching a movie, reading a book or jumping out of an airplane. The key is to find something that works for you and make time to fit that activity into your schedule.

While it is recommended that you take the time to learn more about how stress affects aging and the cycling of hormones to understand the importance of stress reduction in both the body and the eyes, it is more important for you to take action to reduce this stress.

My Vision Therapy System will alleviate strain in the visual system and prevent it from accumulating. Mental stress must be alleviated using other methods.

For some people, the pressure of time constraints, the total amount of stress, or the number of stressful events may simply be too much to handle with their regular strategies. For those who need new or additional ways to control and reduce stress levels, the following suggestions are made.

Binaural Beat Technology

Thoughts, emotions and behaviors all originate from communications between the neurons within our brain. These communications are synchronized electrical pulses from masses of neurons which produce brainwaves. Brainwaves have different frequencies and are measured in hertz (cycles per second). They are divided into bands of slow, moderate, and fast waves, and change according to what we are doing and how we are feeling.

1. Delta waves are generated in the deepest of meditation states and in dreamless sleep. Healing and rejuvenation of the body are stimulated in this state which is the reason why deep restorative sleep is so essential to the body's healing process (0.5 to 3 Hz).

2. Theta waves occur most often in sleep. They also occur during deep mediation. This state is the gateway to learning and memory. We normally only experience this wave state as we wake or drift off to sleep. This is the state where we are able to use the brain's subconscious ability that lies beyond our normal conscious awareness (3 to 8 Hz).

3. Alpha waves occur while we are awake during quiet flowing thoughts that are not quite meditative. Alpha waves are the resting state for the brain and will aid overall mental coordination, calmness, alertness, mind/body integration and learning (8 to 12 Hz).

4. Beta waves dominate our normal waking state of consciousness when attention is directed towards cognitive tasks and things in the world outside our bodies. Beta is a "fast" activity, present when we are alert and attentive, and engaged in problem solving, judgment, decision making, or in focused mental activity. Higher

hertz Beta waves can produce anxiety in the average person. Beta brainwaves are further divided into three bands. Low Beta or Beta 1 (12-15Hz) waves occur during "fast idle" thought. Beta or Beta 2 (15-22Hz) waves occur during high engagement thought. High Beta or Beta 3 (22-38Hz) waves are present during highly complex thought, or based on the person, high anxiety, excitement, agitation, or paranoia. Beta 3 waves are present in a high frequency processing state that takes a tremendous amount of energy to operate in. Beta 3 waves are not a very efficient way for the brain to function.

5. Gamma waves at the low end of the frequency range of 38 - 42Hz are associated with highly complex thought in some people. The average person does not usually produce these types of brain waves under normal circumstances. Similar to High Beta waves, Gamma waves in this range and at higher hertz levels usually produce high anxiety, excitement, agitation, or paranoia in most people unless the individual knows how to utilize and harness them. Highly complex thought at the low end of this higher frequency range 38 - 42Hz, is possible but does not occur often in most people as the waves are hard to produce and utilize effectively. These waves do occur during highly complex thought in very intelligent people at the high genius level and they can produce very high cognitive functioning. Some brainwave scales do not include Gamma waves and extend the Beta 3 range to 42 Hz. (38 to 100 Hz).

It is possible for High Beta or Gamma waves to be utilized for higher cognitive thought if one knows how to utilize and harness the brainwaves at the stated hertz levels. Very few people are able to utilize the waves at the stated hertz levels though, so High Beta or Gamma waves are usually present during periods of mental stress and anguish. If the brainwave frequency that is present during the stress period is changed, the mood of a person's conscious state will also change.

Is changing or altering a brainwave possible?

Brainwaves can be changed in a multitude of ways. Activities such as physical exercise can alter brainwaves. Chemical interventions such as recreational drugs will alter brainwaves. Biofeedback can be used to change brainwaves. Through *resonance*, other frequency waves presented to the brain will also change brainwaves. Simply put, resonance occurs when one object with a vibrating frequency causes a second object to vibrate with the same frequency.

Frequencies can be presented to the brain in many different ways. If two different frequencies are presented separately to your brain from the left and right sides simultaneously, your brain will detect the phase variation between the frequencies and try to reconcile that difference. As the two frequencies mesh in and out of phase with each other, your brain will create its own third signal which is called a binaural beat. The binaural beat is equal to the difference between the two frequencies. If a frequency of 100 Hz is presented to your brain through your left ear, and a frequency of 105 Hz is presented to your brain through your right ear, your brain "hears" and resonates to a third frequency pulsing at 5 Hz, the exact difference between the two frequencies. Research has shown that brain waves will start resonating with a binaural beat, meaning your brainwaves will match that beat or wave. This is called "frequency following response," and it will put brainwaves into the binaural beat wave frequency.

The brainwave created will produce the associated effect that naturally occurs during that brainwave frequency, and can result in relaxation state or stimulative concentrative learning states.

Binaural beat technology has been approved by doctors and scientists around the world. By introducing certain sounds or electrical frequencies to your brain through each ear, you can achieve powerful states of deep relaxation or focused concentration. Binaural beat therapy has been used to induce various brain wave states to treat anxiety and stress, and promote relaxation as well as sleep.

There are many products available with binaural beat technology.

Holosync

The Holosync meditation products by Centerpointe are recommended. Centerpointe technology has been is scientifically proven and is extremely effective in reducing stress as well as increasing intellectual capacity. There is no relationship monetarily or otherwise between the author and Centerpointe.

Holosync Meditation Products by Centerpointe can be found at: www.centerpointe.com.

As Centerpointe products can be cost prohibitive, there are many free binaural beat generators that you can use to create your own binaural beats audio. Binaural beats are best used with a masking music track. When selecting a masking music background track, you should choose an audio track that is relaxing such as falling rain, thunderstorm, trickling creek, ocean waves, classical music, or something else that is calming and that will not captivate or direct your thought. Use any search engine to search for "binaural beat generators."

Sota Bio Tuner

Another option for changing brain waves is the Sota Bio Tuner. Similar to the action of binaural beats, the Sota Bio Tuner uses a broad range of harmonic frequencies generated through electrical impulses and delivered through the ear to alter brainwaves. The result is an enhanced well being and a state of relaxation. The technology can also increase intelligence.

More information on the Bio Tuner can be found at the following links. There is no relationship monetarily or otherwise between this Author and Sota.

www.sota.com

Want More?

I am very grateful that you took the time to read my book.

If you like what you have read and would like even more information about improving your vision, please go to my website and sign up for my email list.

You will be the first to know about new articles; you will receive additional vision therapy techniques and exercises, special offers, and alerts of any new editions and releases of this book.

Here is the link to my website where you can subscribe to my email list:

www.ImproveYourVision.org

I also post information and articles to my Facebook page located at:

https://www.facebook.com/ImproveYourVision

If you enjoyed my book please consider giving me a positive review if available at your selected point of purchase.

Thank you,

Dean Liguori

Author Vision Therapy: Exercise Your Eyes and Improve Your Eyesight

Vision Therapy System

Disclaimer: Before you start this or any vision therapy program, you should get a check up and approval from your eye doctor. There are some rare conditions that could cause your eyes to be further strained or possibly even incur further damage.

Directions

Vision therapy should be performed without wearing any visual correction. If you can focus at all or at least minimally without your glasses, it is recommended that you remove them prior to performing these exercises. If you wear contacts you should remove them before performing the exercises or they could fold or become dislodged. You should try to see throughout the day as much as possible without correction or by trying to use a weaker prescription.

In all cases where correction creates clear eyesight, seeing clearly is merely a matter of adjusting the focal point of light at the proper place on the retina. Vision therapy will train your visual system to do this better.

You may "feel" the ciliary muscles in the eye being worked while performing these exercises. You should also be able to feel the ciliary muscles relax, tension being relieved in the eye, and experience visual clarity returning.

If you are doing these exercises in an attempt to restore damaged vision due to prolonged use of visual correction such as eyeglasses or contact lenses, or disease, it is recommended that you perform the exercises you select in a session at least twice a day, and each individual exercise more times than suggested. You should try to perform some of the exercises for a few minutes throughout the day. Try to perform all of the exercises in this program at some set interval, such as weekly, or regularly rotate through all of the provided exercises rather than only focusing only on the favorites that you develop.

Print the eye charts included in this program to gauge the improvement of your visual acuity. Place the chart on a wall and find the distance from the chart where both eyes can read the first and second lines of type clearly. Mark this point and be sure to stand in the same spot when testing your visual improvement in the future. Test your visual acuity before starting the exercise program. Re-test your visual acuity after the exercises and on a weekly basis, or at any other follow up time interval you choose. Eye charts can also be printed larger than the standard paper size of 8.5 x 11, such as 8.5 x 14, on most printers. Specialty printers can print even larger sizes if needed.

1. Perform all exercises at least a couple times to become familiar with them. Identify which exercises or enjoy or challenge you the most or that provide the most improvement.

2. *Perform these exercises slowly and rhythmically until you get them down. You must follow these guidelines or you will not receive the full benefits of the exercises!*

3. Practicing these exercises often will increase your ability to relax your eye muscles better, and complete these exercises faster.

4. It is better to do these exercises more often and regularly for shorter periods of time verses once in a while for longer periods of time. When you are reading or looking at a

computer screen for extended periods, 30-120 seconds three times every hour, is more beneficial than 5 minutes every couple hours.

5. When the exercise instructs you to move your eye around in its socket, it is important to get the highest range of motion that is possible i.e. try to move your eye as far left/right, up/down, as it will go in your eye socket without moving your head.

6. During each exercise, it is important to focus your vision as best as possible in every direction that you look. Try to maintain focus during the full range of movement. Focus on and see objects in view as your view is moving past them. It is important that you try to focus on the objects that come into view when your eyes by pass them while you perform the exercises. Perform the exercises more slowly if you have problems focusing during them. As your ability to focus increases, you will be able to perform the exercises faster.

7. If you have differences in visual acuity in either eye, cover one eye, and perform exercises in the other eye. Do not close the eye that is not exercising. Closing an eye while focusing with the other can temporarily negatively affect the visual acuity in the closed eye when you open it and then attempt to focus with it. The best ways to cover an eye while keeping it open are with your open palm held in front of it, a patch, or uncorrected non-tinted glasses that have one lens covered with a piece of paper. Be sure to exercise both of your eyes if you elect to cover one to exercise it independently of the other. Close one eye and check the clarity of vision through the other eye at different times throughout the day to determine if you have eye dominance issues.

8. Once you perform all of the exercises multiple times, try to pick at least one exercise from each group and perform all of those exercises at least daily. Each group of exercises

targets a different area, and it is recommended that one from each group be used at each exercise session daily. Focus on exercises that are more difficult for you to perform as you are likely to get more improvement from them. You will have favorite exercises, and these will be the ones you will be most likely to perform regularly. You should at least on a weekly basis, perform all of the exercises to test your performance and see the benefit you are receiving. If your vision improvement progress stalls or you are not seeing results, try switching up the exercises. It is not abnormal to experience improvements in your eyesight almost immediately. Do not hesitate to change up the exercises you are using to ensure you continue to get positive results.

9. It is recommended that you perform your vision therapy program for a minimum of 15 minutes per day. You get out of vision therapy what you put in. It is possible to see greater improvement in eyesight when vision therapy is performed more often and for longer periods of time. It is important to take short breaks throughout the day to perform vision therapy, even if only 30-120 seconds, especially when performing tasks that stress your eyesight such as reading or looking at phone or computer screens.

10. Competition sometimes brings out the best in people. Consider beginning vision therapy with a partner, not for performing the exercises, but for the challenge of who can improve their eyesight faster.

11. It is recommended that you keep a journal of your vision therapy sessions. This is especially important if you feel that your eyesight improvement progress is not progressing as fast as you would like. You should perform a vision test before and after each vision therapy session and record it in the journal. You should also include the specific therapy exercises performed, the duration of therapy time, additional

therapy exercises performed throughout the day, and any another notes or things experienced. Use the sample journal provided or come up with your own.

12. Consider seeking out a vision therapy teacher to advise you or help you further customize a personal vision therapy program. To find a board certified vision therapy doctor near you use the "Locate a Doctor" by zip code function on the homepage of the College of Optometrists in Vision Development website (www.covd.org)

Vision Therapy Eye Exercises

The eye exercises are broken up into six (6) groups:

1. Eye Region Massage and Relaxation Exercises
2. Eye Relaxation Exercises
3. Eye Movement Exercises
4. Eye Focusing Exercises
5. Preventing and Correcting Computer Vision Syndrome
6. Hand Eye Coordination Exercises for Improvement in Athletic Performance

The program begins with exercises to relax and reduce stress in and around the eye and progresses to those of rapid focus and quick accommodation. The program progressively moves from relaxation and stress relief to exercises that recondition and strengthen the eyes abilities to quickly focus and accommodate.

Eye Region Massage and Relaxation Exercises

Notes on these exercises

Accommodation and visual acuity is affected by overall body stress as well as accumulated stress in and around the region of the eyes. These exercises, acupressure points, and massage areas, will relieve stress in those areas. Try all of the exercises, and keep the ones that you prefer or that are the most effective for you.

Exercises

1. <u>Temple</u> - Put the tips of your index finger and middle finger of each hand just over the bony ridge above each outer corner of your eye in the temple area. Use the tips of your fingers to gently massage this area. You can massage into the area of the temple as well. If this area is painful it should become less so after you massage. Perform for a count of ten, repeat for three.

2. <u>Inner Cheekbone</u> - Move the tips of your fingers under the inner corners of your eye just below the bone of the eye socket. They should be under the part of the cheekbone where it attaches towards the upper part of the nose. You should feel a slight indentation or depression in the area between the nose and cheekbone. Massage this area gently for a count of ten, repeat three times.

3. Tip of Jawbone - Move your fingers down and outward from the above spot to the lower tip of the cheekbone. Use your fingers or your thumb turned sideways to press on this spot. Work from the front towards the back of the cheekbone where you will feel your jaw muscles. Gently press and release for counts of ten, repeat three times.

4. Jawbone Joint - Place your fingers in front of each ear, then open and shut your mouth. Move your fingers down into the front part of the joint of the jawbone. Massage gently for a count of ten, repeat three times.

5. Back of Jawbone Find the bone just under the lobe of your ear. With your thumb, massage behind this bone and in the area. Repeat twice.

6. Eye Socket Bone - close your eyes and use your index and middle fingers to massage the surrounding bones of both eye sockets. Include the bridge of the nose, and temple areas. repeat for three or as desired

7. Back of Neck behind Ear Lobes - With both hands reach behind the ear on the (same hand side) and using the first three fingers of each hand massage each bone at the side and back of the neck and surrounding areas. repeat for three or as desired

8. "Eyes" Behind the Back of your Head - With both hands as in the previous exercise, follow the same bone up the back of your head towards the top of your head. You will feel indentations on each side of the back of your head almost directly behind the eye sockets. With the same fingers, gently massage these indented areas in the back of the skull directly behind the eyes. They may be very tender.

9. Big Toe - The big toe is a Chinese acupressure point that can improve blood supply to the brain and optic nerves as well as

relax neck muscles. Rotate both of your big toes in clockwise and counterclockwise circles and then massage them thoroughly including the front, back, sides, and top of the toe.

10. Reflex areas on the sole of each foot directly behind the second and third toes - Use the thumb and index finger of either hand to press downward and massage upwards in the areas directly behind the second and third toes on the sole of the foot. Work up and down 8 times per foot and switch. Massage each foot independently. Repeat 3 -8 times.

11. Eyebrow Bone - Place three fingers of each hand on the bone of eyebrow over the eye. The gripping part of the fingers of each hand should be facing the eye. The fingers of your two hands should be about an inch apart as measured between your eyebrows. Gently applying pressure with your eyes closed and slide your fingers down under the eyebrow bone towards your eye to the under part of the eye socket bone. As you are applying pressure to the skin, the skin should move with your fingers as your fingers slide into this position. This means that your fingers do not slide over the skin. You will be applying gentle pressure between the eye socket bone and the eye ball. While doing this it may be more comfortable for you to look down with your eye while your eye is closed. While applying gentle pressure the color in your field of vision should get darker or pure black.

12. Figure Eight head movements - There are many different variations you can use in performing this exercise. It consists of closing your eyes and drawing imaginary figure eights in the air with your nose. Performing smaller circles of figure eights help to relax the eye. Larger circles help to relax the muscles in the head and neck. This exercise can be performed quickly, and can be done anywhere, and anytime your eyes need to relax. If can be done with the eyes open or shut. If you like this exercise, any design can be substituted

in place of the figure eights. Some suggestions include simple circles, writing words in the air, or drawing stars, the options are only limited by your imagination. Use full range of motion.

Eye Relaxation Exercises

1. Palming

Palming was originally a "yoga" technique and relaxes the whole visual system. It was a key component of Dr. Bates' system. Our eyes work by converting light rays into images. If there were no light entering the eye, one would expect there to be an absence of images. However, in stressed eyes or even those with impaired eyesight, swirling patches of colors can and usually appear, creating images and pictures where there should be none. This is a symptom of eyestrain that can cause impaired vision. Palming makes people aware of the presence of eyestrain and the calming touch of the hands helps relax the tension in the eye.

When you start palming you may see swirling colors or gray patches. As you begin to relax, you should notice your visual field becoming blacker to the point of total blackness. You should focus on achieving this blackness. This is a signal that your visual system is relaxing. The goal is to achieve perfect blackness.

Exercise

Place your palms over your closed eyes. It is preferred that your fingers cross over at the forehead but you can keep them straight. You can also use the "meaty" part of the palm for this exercise or your slightly cupped hands. The exact position of your palms is up to you. Be careful to not press or apply pressure on the eyeballs. This will put pressure on the blood vessels in the eyeballs and reduce circulation of blood and nutrients. Do not cover or block your nose. You may rest your elbows on a table surface as long as you are not putting pressure on your eyes from your palms; if necessary support the weight of your head with your fingers on your forehead. Try to block as much light as possible with your palms. Put yourself in a comfortable and proper posture while palming. Keep your eyes closed behind your palms. Concentrate on deep breathing, the most important thing to do in this exercise is to relax your vision and eyes. Try to imagine pleasant scenery such as floating clouds in a blue sky, a sunrise, mountains, or the sea. Prior to palming, if it helps you to relax, you may rub your hands together until they are warm before you cover your eyes. You can perform the palming relaxation method for as long as you would like, or until you see total blackness. It is recommended that you do it for at least three minutes.

2. Controlling your Focus

Notes on this exercise

This exercise teaches you to manually control the focus of your eye. You are manually controlling the ciliary muscle when you perform this exercise. This relaxes the ciliary muscle and improves accommodation. Quick accommodation at varied distances allows the ciliary muscles to relax and loosen up, and the lens to relax into an unconstricted shape. It can and should be done together and individually where the other eye is covered. You will get the most benefit performing this exercise outdoors or in front of a window.

Exercise

Open your eyes as wide as possible and let your vision go out of focus. You may have to concentrate to take your vision out of focus. This is best done by letting your vision completely relax to the point that you are not focusing or out of focus. This is what happens when you close your eyes, yet in this circumstance you keep your eye lids open. When you do this properly you may experience a type of "double vision." Once you get use to making this or allowing this to happen, it will become easier to do. Once you let your vision go out of focus, bring it back in focus on a particular object. Repeat this with different objects at different distances, both near and far.

Eye Movement Exercises

Notes on these exercises:

These exercises are not just for the muscles around the eye that move the eye back and forth; they also teach the ciliary muscles to accommodate during movement. For this reason it is important to focus during the movement of the eye to force the eye to jump from object to object at different distances while crossing a plane. It is also important to stretch the field of view at the edges and limits of your peripheral vision.

You may get a better result doing these in a larger room with varied distances between objects, in front of a window, or outside.

Exercises

1. Moving both eyes in a straight line - Move eyes up and down 10 times, then side to side 10 times. Repeat 2 more times. Do not move your head. Focus on objects as they cross the visual plane and you move your field of vision.

2. Rotating both eyes in a circular motion - Move eyes in a circle clockwise 10 times, then counterclockwise for 10 circles. Repeat 2 more times. Do not move your head. Focus on objects as they cross the visual plane as you move your field of vision.

3. Figure Eights - Different than figure eight head movements, these exercises are done with the eyes only while the head is held still. Similar to figure eight head movements, there are

many different variations you can use in performing this exercise. Move eyes in a figure eight pattern clockwise 10 times, then counterclockwise for 10 circles. Repeat 2 more times. Do not move your head. Focus on objects as they cross the visual plane. Performing larger circles allow the eye to accommodate at larger distances and a greater range of motion in the eye socket. As with head movements, any design can be substituted in place of the figure eights; suggestions include writing words in the air, or drawing stars, etc., the options are only limited by your imagination.

Eye Focusing Exercises

Notes on these exercises:

Focusing exercises performed quickly between different varied distances teaches better accommodation and increases the ability to manually and automatically focus on objects.

Exercises

1. Farsight/Nearsight focus drills: This exercise requires you to quickly focus between a close object and a far object. Find an object that is between 6 inches and 18 inches from your nose, and another object that is further away at a distance you can focus on at the limit of your visual field or as far as your office or window will allow. Make sure that the first object does not block the view of the second object. You might have to look in a different direction, or reposition yourself to find an object. Focus on the closer object and then quickly switch your focus to the further object. Keep shifting your focus back and forth between the objects. Be sure to acquire a good focus on each object before switching to the other. Increase the speed at which you can pull the different objects into focus and switch. If you are doing this right (maybe after much practicing) you should be able to feel the ciliary muscle being worked. Switch your focus 10 times, and repeat twice. For those who have differences in accommodation or visual acuity between eyes, this exercise can be done with one eye at a time, cover the other with your hand and leave that eye open. If you have trouble seeing without correction, pick targets that you can focus on clearly and every time you

perform this exercise attempt to increase or decrease the distances at which you can focus.

Variations:

    a. Stand in front of a window and place a dot or a sticker on the window and use this as your near target

    b. As you get better at bringing these objects into focus, add a third or fourth target at different distances and switch between them. Try to go back and forth from near to far.

    c. Instead of using a fixed target as your near point use a pen. Hold the pen at arm's length in front of you. While keeping it in focus, slowly bring it towards your nose until you can no longer focus on it clearly. Move the pen back until you regain focus on it. At this point switch your view to your more distant target. Keep the pen at a smaller range of motion where you can take it in and out of focus quickly. You can also try to push the boundaries of focus for the pen both near and far. Study the smallest details on the pen while it is going in and out of focus to increase your visual acuity. You can perform this variation with one eye and with multiple targets.

    d. Use one eye at a time, covering the other.

2. <u>Double object focus:</u> In this exercise, you can use the same objects as before. You will attempt to focus on both of the objects at the same time. This is done by identifying, and focusing on, an imaginary point between the objects. This exercise is harder to perform because there is no "real" object to focus on, you must pick, and focus, at a point between

your objects, which will allow you to keep both of them fairly clearly. You must find this imaginary point that will allow both objects to be seen and when you find it you will be looking at the imaginary point directly. *You will not be looking at either of your objects directly*, you will see them in almost "peripheral" vision. The closest object will be slightly beneath the imaginary point; the furthest object will be slightly above the imaginary point. You will have to concentrate on focusing at the imaginary point to see both objects. This exercise might take some practice. Like the previous exercise, you should be able to feel the ciliary muscle working. You should use this exercise with one eye at a time as well.

Variations:

    a. To start out in making this exercise easier if you need to, you can use three objects at varying distances while focusing on the object in the middle. The goal of the exercise is not to focus on a specific target but at nothing, thereby helping you to learn to manually adjust the focus of your eyes automatically.

    b. Add a third target and attempt to slightly shift the focal point to balance your focus on all three objects.

    c. Pick near and far targets that are not directly in line but that have some distance in width, left and right or high and low, between them. This will also cause you to focus across a plane as well at a distance variation. Be sure to switch what sides the near and far targets are on.

    d. Use one eye at a time, covering the other.

3. <u>Shifting of Focus Far to Near</u>: With both eyes open find a far point or object and focus on it. While focusing on the object, position your finger or a pen about 6-12 inches in front of your face. Whether your finger or a pen is used, you should see two of them. Switch your focus to your finger or pen and you will see two of the object that you were previously focusing on. Switch your views back and forth after focusing on the fine details of the object. Repeat this 10 times. This exercise helps correct the dominance of one eye over the other in sight. It relieves accumulated stress on your eyes, restores elasticity of the ciliary muscles and lens, and improves your ability to focus. This is a great exercise to use for quick breaks while engaging in activities such as reading or viewing computer screens. You must use both eyes for this exercise.

4. <u>Thumbing</u>: Stretch out your arm in front of you with your thumb pointed up in the "thumbs up" or "hitchhike" position. Put your visual focus on your thumb as your arm is outstretched. Bring your thumb closer to you, while maintaining focus, until your thumb is about 3 inches in front of your face. Move your thumb away until your arm is fully outstretched, again maintaining focus the entire time. You can vary the speed and lengths of your arm movements to change up this exercise. Try this exercise with one eye at a time, covering the other eye with your non moving hand.

5. <u>Yardstick, Stick, or String Exercise #1</u>: This exercise requires the assistance of a straight object. A stick or string approximately 3 feet in length is ideal for this exercise. Stand or sit about six feet from a wall. Vertically hold the stick about a foot from your nose with one end pointing at the floor, and the other at the ceiling. Focus up and down the stick, from the bottom to the top and vice versa. Focus up and back down 10 times. Now focus up and down the wall, from the bottom to the top and vice versa. Focus up and down 10 times. While looking up and down the wall the stick should seem to

become two sticks side by side. Repeat this entire set three or four times. On different days of performing this exercise, alternate the distances between the wall and your seat.

6. Yardstick, Stick, or Ruler Exercise #2: This exercise requires the assistance of a hard straight object. A stick approximately 3 feet in length is ideal for this exercise, although a long ruler can substitute. Horizontally hold the stick about three inches from your nose, with one end pointing at your nose and the other at the wall. Focus up and down the stick, from the nearest point on the stick to the farthest point and vice versa. When you are looking at the nearest or farthest end of the stick, you should see a "V." When you are moving your eyes between the ends of the stick, you should see an "X." If, when you are looking at the ends of the stick you see a "Y" instead of a "V," one eye is weaker than the other. To strengthen the weaker eye's accommodation, cover the stronger eye with your hand and focus the weaker eye up and down the stick by itself. This exercise will improve the eye's ability to accommodate. When the weaker eye gets stronger and you look down the yardstick with both eyes the bottom of the "Y" will get shorter and shorter, until it disappears. If you see a "V" upon starting this exercise, focus up and down the stick 10 times, and repeat three times.

7. Horizontal movement object focus Exercise: While riding as a passenger in a moving vehicle, look out of the window of the vehicle at as much of a 90 degree angle as possible. Your goal is to focus on a passing object clearly and then switch to another one as soon as you get the object in focus. You should be constantly switching your focus to a new object as soon as you focus clearly on the current one. The ideal distance should be between 10 and 25 feet, this distance will vary based on the speed of the vehicle and your ability of your eyes to be able to accommodate objects. The speed of the vehicle should be a minimum of 35 mph. At slower

distances try to focus at closer distances. At faster speeds you may have to focus to a farther distance. If it is difficult for you to focus on closer objects, pick ones that are farther away. Work to be able to improve your focus by moving to closer objects, as they move past your visual field much more quickly. Try not to move your head, only your eyes as you move your eyes and shift focus to quickly passing objects. As you get better and switch your view quickly at closer objects, this may become more difficult, but you should try to keep your head moving as little as possible. Your eyes will have to fix on and track an object for a split second to gain focus before you have to immediately jump to the next object to focus. After a pause to gain focus, it should feel like your eyes jump forward to lock on the next object. You will have to use your peripheral vision to find the next object. Things to focus on can simply be objects on the ground such as a grass clump, weed, bush, rock, a sign, piece of garbage, or pole. Signs with writing that you can attempt to read or discern the letters on are good objects. You can choose to switch focus between objects that are high then low, or large and small. The goal is to be able to accommodate smaller objects closer to the vehicle at faster speeds. Switch the sides of the vehicle that you look out of. Once you get use to this exercise, you may find that is best performed on the expressway in the city where the focal points are 10-25 feet away and you are traveling between 55 and 75 mph. Seek to shorten distances or increase the speed at which you can accommodate. You can also perform this exercise with one eye at a time. This is a fun and challenging exercise.

8. <u>Rotating Object Focus Exercise:</u> Although it is more difficult to find a device to work with for this exercise, it is very fun and effective. Find something that is fixated in one place or one point, and rotates; a ceiling fan or record on record player are good choices. Tape printed letters or pictures of various sizes at different positions on the rotating device. Be

sure to have different sized letters and pictures, and have them equally spread out around the part of the device that rotates i.e. close to the center spinning point, towards the edges, and in the space between. While the object is rotating fixate on one object and keep it in focus for 1-3 seconds, then switch to another object and repeat. Perform this exercise for periods of 1-5 minutes. Vary the viewing distance and the rotating speeds. If using a ceiling fan the best place to perform the exercise it to lay on a couch or the floor directly under the taped objects.

9. Patch therapy: Cover one eye and focus out of the other at an object close to the furthest limits of your visual range. If vision is blurry in the eye you are looking out of, or it is uncomfortable to focus, you may have eye dominance. Test both eyes. Do not close one eye while doing this; instead cover it with your hand. If you have an eye that is dominant or lazy, you can train the weaker eye to become more dominant by covering the dominant eye and performing normal daily activities such as reading with it, working on the computer, watching TV, etc. Do not perform any dangerous activity or anything else that requires depth perception such as driving while one eye is covered. This is called patch therapy. It is normal for an optometrist or an ophthalmologist to recommend this exercise for children, but not adults even though it is very beneficial for all. The best way to cover the dominant eye is with a patch or non-corrective no tint glasses that have one lens covered with tape or paper. Slightly tinted glasses or those with color such as yellow tint can also be used. This treatment may make you feel weird or off balance when walking after you cover the eye or when you uncover the eye. When you uncover the dominant eye it is not unusual to notice a substantial improvement in combined visual acuity. If you do not have a dominant eye or if you also need to improve the vision in your dominant eye as well, you can perform this exercise with each eye individually as it

helps train each eye to accommodate better individually. If you have a dominant eye, spend more time with that eye covered to reduce the dominance. You can also use the patch to perform other eye exercises.

10. Pinhole Glasses Exercise: This exercise helps to strengthen your eye's ability to accommodate. The improvements seen while putting these glasses on can also indicate the visual acuity that vision therapy can help you improve to. You can use smaller objects in or close to the perimeter of your visual range of clarity, or the vision chart provided. Position yourself at the proper distance from the object you choose. Put your pinhole glasses on and focus on a hole in the pinhole glasses for about 3 seconds. Switch your focus though the pinhole to the object for about 10 seconds. Shift your focus back to any hole of your glasses, and maintain focus for 3 seconds. Repeat this process for 5 to 10 minutes daily. Your eyes could become "tired" after performing this exercise. It is important that you follow this exercise with a relaxation exercise such as palming for at least 3-5 minutes. Attempt to push or lengthen the distance of your visual perimeter when repeating this exercise from day to day. Improvement in this exercise will be seen through shortened time to switch your focus back and forth from near to far objects.

The Following Eye Exercises Specifically Target Nearsightedness and Farsightedness

Sight field variation exercise for those with Presbyopia or who are far-sighted:

> You will need a paragraph of text or an object with print on it. With both eyes open while holding the object, move it away from your eyes until you can see it very clearly. Move the object slightly closer until it begins to blur, and then back to its starting position. Move the object backwards and forwards across your point of clear vision. As you continue to perform this movement you should notice that you are able to move the object closer to achieve the same visual blur. Once you can view the writing on the object clearly at about 6 inches you can find an object with smaller print and repeat the exercise. With eye dominance issues this exercise can be repeated with one eye closed.

Sight field variation exercise for those with Myopia or who are near-sighted:

> You will need a paragraph of text or an object with print on it. While covering one eye, hold the object in the other hand and move it away from you. Once you find the furthest point that your open eye can see clearly, move the object closer and then backwards and forwards across your point of clear vision. Doing this will improve and extend your ability to focus. Repeat the exercise for your covered eye. You can also try this exercise with both eyes.

Preventing and Correcting Computer Vision Syndrome

Much can be done to reduce the occurrence of Computer Vision Syndrome. Controlling and changing the type of workplace lighting, preventing glare, adjusting screen contrast and resolution, establishing and varying proper working distances, and maintaining good posture for computer viewing, are ways to help minimize the symptoms of Computer Vision Syndrome.

Visual practices to help prevent CVS include blinking more frequently. Those who work on computers for extended periods have been found to blink about five times less than average. Blinking less frequently causes tears to evaporate more quickly and leads to dryer eyes. Those who blink slowly 10 times every 20 minutes re-moisturize their eyes.

Eyestrain and focusing fatigue occurs when one focuses at close distances like a computer screen for too long. The 20-20-20 rule helps prevent eyestrain. The 20-20-20 rule calls for one to look away from the screen at an object that is at least 20 feet away, every 20 minutes, for 20 seconds. Another way to relieve accumulated stress from building up in the ciliary muscles of the eye is to look away from the computer screen at an object that is far away from you for 10 to 15 seconds and then look at a closer object closer to you for 10 to 15 seconds and performing this sequence 10 times. Use objects outside a window if objects at longer distances are needed.

Use a combination of eye focusing exercises in accordance with the 20-20-20 rule. Lengthen the exercise time to 30-120 seconds if necessary to relieve eye tension and restore focus at varied distances.

Combination Exercise for Extensive Reading or Computer Vision Syndrome

Notes on this exercise

These exercises are good to perform when you are reading or looking at computer screens for long periods of time and quickly need to relax or stretch your eyes. Perform these during short breaks while reading or looking at a computer screen for long periods. For the best results, perform portions or parts of the exercise every 10-15 minutes while looking up from your reading material or away from your computer screen at greater distances, otherwise use the 20-20-20 rule.

Exercises

a. Close both of your eyes and hold both of your lids shut. Squeeze your lids tightly closed for 1-5 seconds and open them quickly. Open your eyes as wide as possible arching your brows and stretching your face. Focus on an object at a distance while you are stretching. Repeat one to three times.

b. Blink rapidly a dozen or so times while trying to focus forward on a different distant object between each of the blinks.

c. After Blinking, open your eyes wide and focus on objects using the full range of your visual field by looking up as far as possible and then down as far as possible, without moving your head. Trying to focus at the limits of your visual field around the edges of your visual field is more important than focusing while moving the eye. Do this slowly and as deliberately as possible. To further relax you can combine breathing with the change in direction; inhale on up, and exhale on down. You can move your eyes from left to right, up and down, diagonally, or any other pattern your prefer.

d. Rotate your eyes around the peripheral area of your visual field in a circle without moving your head. Try to focus on objects at and beyond what your visual field allows around your entire eye. Try to focus at the limits of your visual field around the edges of your visual field. Do this slowly and as deliberately as possible. You can try to do this with one eye at a time, or with both. Attempt to stretch your focus beyond what your visual field will allow and go around the eye 6-12 times. Be sure to switch directions half way through the exercise; do not rotate your eyes in the same direction for the whole exercise.

e. Focus outside a window at an object located at the furthest distance of your visual range until that object becomes clear. Know what the normal furthest distance of your visual range is and keep focusing out to objects in that range until clear vision returns at that range. Cover one eye and focus with the other to ensure that the ability to focus in each eye improves equally.

Hand Eye Coordination Exercises for Improvement in Athletic Performance

The sharpness of visual acuity and speed of accommodation have major impacts in athletic performance. The ability to coordinate visual acuity and accommodation with body movements is crucial to athletic performance in many sports.

Exercise and Notes

Ball Bounce against Wall: This exercise is simply bouncing a ball against the wall and catching it. A tennis ball, racquetball, rubber ball, etc. can be used. It is recommended that you start with a larger slower ball such as a tennis ball and as your performance improves gradually move towards using faster balls such as the racquetball and ultimately a very fast moving smaller sized hard rubber ball. The harder that the rubber ball is, the faster your reaction time will need to be. As one variation gets easy, move to a harder variation and then to a smaller and faster moving ball. Do not discount the benefits of this exercise with its variations to improve your visual acuity, accommodation and hand eye coordination with body movement.

Exercise and Variations

Ball Bounce against Wall

1. Both Eyes: with both eyes open perform the following:

    a. Both Hands: bounce the ball against the wall using both hands to catch. Use either your left or right hand as needed to throw and catch. Progress towards using both hands to throw and catch equally. Progress to throwing the ball from the side that it is caught. This would mean that you might be throwing the ball with a backhand depending on which hand and side the ball was caught on i.e. left hand catch on the right side would require a backhand throw. Strive to use both hands equally. Move your feet as needed to catch and throw the ball. Use freedom of movement both laterally and in and out from the wall.

b. <u>Alternate Both Hands</u>: same as above but with the goal of catching and throwing while alternating between your left and right hand. Use freedom of movement both laterally and in and out from the wall.

c. <u>One Hand</u>: Same as (a) but using only one hand to catch and throw. Progress towards catching and throwing with the same one left or right hand, alternating between catching and throwing on your left then right sides. Switch hands for equal throws. Use freedom of movement both laterally and in and out from the wall.

d. <u>Standing on One Leg</u>: Perform the same variations listed above while standing on one leg. Attempt to stand on one leg while catching and throwing the ball. Doing this will require you to shift your hips around, as well as the foot that you are standing on from side to side, depending on the required movements. If you need to use both feet to stabilize yourself to catch the ball, do so, but go back to standing on one foot to throw the ball. In order to stand on one foot, the ball will need to be both thrown and caught in a tighter pattern. Try to reduce the times that you need to go to both feet to move in order to catch the ball. You may also bounce around on one leg to use freedom of movement both laterally and in and out from the wall.

2. One Eye: with one eye open and the other covered, perform the following variations. Do not just close one eye to use the other; it is highly recommended to use a patch to cover the eye to improve performance. If you do not have any other way to cover one eye you can close it. If you have trouble seeing the ball with only one eye you may open the closed eye as needed to cheat until your performance improves and you are able to use only one eye to perform effectively. Use the same variations as provided for both eyes open.

   a. Both Hands: bounce the ball against the wall using both hands to catch. Use either your left or right hand as needed to throw and catch. Progress towards using both hands to throw and catch equally. Progress to throwing the ball from the side that it is caught. This would mean that you might be throwing the ball with a backhand depending on which hand and side the ball was caught on i.e. left hand catch on the right side would require a backhand throw. Strive to use both hands equally. Move your feet as needed to catch and throw the ball. Use freedom of movement both laterally and in and out from the wall.

   b. Alternate Both Hands: same as above but with the goal of catching and throwing while alternating between your left and right hand. Use freedom of movement both laterally and in and out from the wall.

c. <u>One Hand</u>: Same as (a) but using only one hand to catch and throw. Progress towards catching and throwing with the same one left or right hand, alternating between catching and throwing on your left then right sides. Switch hands for equal throws. Use freedom of movement both laterally and in and out from the wall.

d. <u>Standing on One Leg</u>: Perform the same variations listed above while standing on one leg. Attempt to stand on one leg while catching and throwing the ball. Doing this will require you to shift your hips around, as well as the foot that you are standing on from side to side, depending on the required movements. If you need to use both feet to stabilize yourself to catch the ball, do so, but go back to standing on one foot to throw the ball. In order to stand on one foot, the ball will need to be both thrown and caught in a tighter pattern. Try to reduce the times that you need to go to both feet to move in order to catch the ball. You may also bounce around on one leg to use freedom of movement both laterally and in and out from the wall. Alternate between the eyes that are closed; close your left eye and stand on your left leg, and close your left eye while standing on your right leg. This is important because different sides of the brain control the left and right functions of the body.

Exercise Tips

1. Your eyes shift about 80 times a second; this helps to keep your ciliary muscles from getting stiff. Staring at anything impedes this natural relaxation. This is especially true when you are watching TV. Shutting your eyes and blinking frequently helps your eyes to relax.

2. Remember to try to fully focus your eyes during any eye movement exercises.

3. Try not to keep any reading material too close to your eyes. Vary the reading distances while reading, studying, or looking at computer screens for extended periods. This will allow your ciliary muscles to hold the lens in slightly different positions.

4. While reading, let your eyes glide easily over the text without straining. Look up from the text now and then to glance around the room. Take a break from your work consistently every 10-15 minutes and focus on objects at varying distances or perform some of these exercises, or follow the 20-20-20 rule. If your vision is blurry at distances where it is otherwise clear when you look up from your reading material, it is recommended that you take breaks more often and perform your selected eye exercises for relief more frequently. You can pick a few favorite exercises or parts of exercises to perform for 10-120 seconds between reading intervals that you determine necessary.

5. It is better to do these exercises for a shorter time regularly, than once in a while for longer periods of time. Performing these exercises 30-60 seconds every hour while you are talking on the phone or waiting on your computer at work, is very beneficial.

6. Choose your favorite exercises or ones that work for you and perform them regularly. Rotate through all exercises at a set interval of time. If you do not see immediate results, be persistent. Remember that it may have taken years for your eyes to weaken. A majority of people experience vision improvement while completing eye exercises. Even though it should not take weeks or months for you to notice some visual acuity improvement, you may not be able to notice results immediately upon performing or completing the exercises.

7. To help improve your vision or eliminate your need for corrective visual devices, you need to try to see without the aid of your corrective glasses as often as you can. It would be better to discard them for longer periods of time if possible. The best time to do this is after your eye exercises. Leave your glasses off for as long as it is comfortable to do so. Another suggestion is to buy weaker eyeglass prescriptions. Try to wear these lower prescription glasses as often as you can. Again, do this for as long as it is comfortable for you to do so. The goal is to completely eliminate your dependence on corrective lenses. Many people find that using their normal prescription becomes painful to their eyes as their vision improves and they must go to a weaker prescription or go without correction for longer periods of time, or for more daily tasks.

References

1. American Optometric Association http://www.aoa.org, "Definition of Optometric Vision Therapy," http://www.aoa.org/Documents/optometrists/QI/definition-of-optometric-vision-therapy.pdf

2. American Optometric Association, "Vision Therapy," http://www.aoa.org/optometrists/education-and-training/clinical-care/vision-therapy?sso=y

3. American Association for Pediatric Ophthalmology, "Vision Therapy," www.aapos.org/terms/conditions/108

4. College of Optometrists in Vision Development (COVD), "Certification." https://covd.site-ym.com/?page=Certification&hhSearchTerms=%22board+and+certification%22 - If link is broken, go to http://www.covd.org/, and search for board certification.

5. About Leonard J. Press, FCOVD, FAAO, "Meet Dr. Leonard Press," http://www.pressvision.com/about_family_eyecare_associates.php

6. Interview by Rachel Cooper of Optometrists Network with Leonard J. Press, FCOVD, FAAO http://www.visiontherapy.org/vision-therapy/faqs/vision-therapy-FAQs.html

7. The Vision Council, "Subject Matter Experts'" http://www.thevisioncouncil.org/subject-matter-experts

8. GlassesCrafter.com, "What Percentage of the Population Wears Glasses?" http://glassescrafter.com/information/percentage-population-wears-glasses.html

9. Dr. William H. Bates, M. D "The Cure of Imperfect Eyesight by Treatment Without Glasses"

10. Wikipedia, "Cushing's Disease/Syndrome," https://en.wikipedia.org/wiki/Cushing%27s_syndrome

11. GlassesCrafter.com, "What Percentage of the Population Wears Glasses?" http://glassescrafter.com/information/percentage-population-wears-glasses.html

12. Mayo Clinic, "Lazy eye (amblyopia)," http://www.mayoclinic.org/diseases-conditions/lazy-eye/basics/definition/con-20029771

13. Gary Heiting OD, All About Vision, "How Contacts Work" http://www.allaboutvision.com/contacts/faq/how-contacts-work.htm

14. American Optometric Association, "Computer Vision Syndrome Symptoms" http://www.aoa.org/optometrists/tools-and-resources/clinical-care-publications/environmentaloccupational-vision/computer-use-needs/computer-vision-syndrome-symptoms?sso=y

15. Non GMO Project, "GMO Facts Frequently asked questions," http://www.nongmoproject.org/learn-more/

16. Non GMO Project, "GMO Facts Frequently asked questions," http://www.nongmoproject.org/learn-more/

17. CBS News, "Study on genetically modified corn, herbicide and tumors reignites controversy," http://www.cbsnews.com/news/study-on-genetically-modified-corn-herbicide-and-tumors-reignites-controversy/

18. www.PubMed.gov, "Life-span exposure to low doses of aspartame beginning during prenatal life increases cancer effects in rats," http://www.ncbi.nlm.nih.gov/pubmed/17805418

19. Natural Society, "Aspartame Exposed – GM Bacteria Used to Create Deadly Sweetener," http://naturalsociety.com/aspartame-exposed-gm-bacteria-used-to-create-deadly-sweetener/

20. Elephant Journal, "Sneaky Names for MSG: Check Your Labels," http://www.elephantjournal.com/2013/04/sneaky-names-for-msg-check-your-labels/

21. "The Truth about Aspartame, MSG and Excitotoxins, An interview with Dr. Russell Blaylock," Dr. Russel Blaylock

22. World Health Organization, "10 Facts on Physical Activity" Updated February 2014, http://www.who.int/features/factfiles/physical_activity/en/

23. The World Health Organization, "Global Recommendations on Physical Activity for Health," http://www.who.int/dietphysicalactivity/factsheet_adults/en/

24. www.PubMed.gov "Hormone profiles in humans experiencing military survival training" https://www.ncbi.nlm.nih.gov/pubmed/10807962?dopt=Abstract

25. Life Extension Magazine, "Reducing the Risks of High Cortisol'" http://www.lef.org/Magazine/2011/9/Reducing-the-Risks-of-High-Cortisol/Page-01

Vision Therapy Journal

Vision Therapy Journal

Name: _____

Week of: _____

Exercises for the week:

1 _____
2 _____
3 _____
4 _____
5 _____
6 _____
7 _____
8 _____
9 _____
10 _____

Day or Session	Start Test Chart / Line / # Correct	Duration in minutes	End Test Chart / Line / # Correct
1	___ / ___ / ___	_____	___ / ___ / ___
2	___ / ___ / ___	_____	___ / ___ / ___
3	___ / ___ / ___	_____	___ / ___ / ___
4	___ / ___ / ___	_____	___ / ___ / ___
5	___ / ___ / ___	_____	___ / ___ / ___
6	___ / ___ / ___	_____	___ / ___ / ___
7	___ / ___ / ___	_____	___ / ___ / ___

Notes:

_____
_____
_____
_____

Eye Charts

These charts can copied and enlarged or they can be downloaded in color at:

http://improveyourvision.org/eye-chart-download/

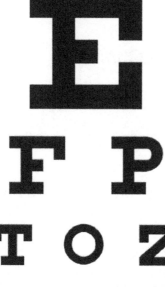

1	20/200
2	20/100
3	20/70
4	20/50
5	20/40
6	20/30
7	20/25
8	20/20
9	
10	
11	

ƎMEW — $\frac{20}{100}$

MƎEME — $\frac{20}{80}$

WMEƎWƎ — $\frac{20}{60}$

EWMƎMEM — $\frac{20}{50}$

ƎEWMEWE — $\frac{20}{40}$

EMƎWƎMƎ — $\frac{20}{30}$

MEWƎWMƎ — $\frac{20}{25}$

WEWMƎEW — $\frac{20}{20}$

EWMƎEMM — $\frac{20}{16}$

70 ft - 21 m	A
	Z Y
60 ft - 18 m	
50 ft - 15 m	E U W Q
40 ft - 12 m	M N D H R
30 ft - 9 m	E Y L U Z M
20 ft - 6 m	R K E X E X A R
15 ft - 4.5 m	W V X P B Z S U W G

70 ft – 21 m	J
60 ft – 18 m	L Y
50 ft – 15 m	W H H H
40 ft – 12 m	B Y V A N
30 ft – 9 m	T N H Q W E
20 ft – 6 m	I Y C C Y U K Z
15 ft – 4.5 m	J M M S Y D G R H M

70 ft – 21 m	T
60 ft – 18 m	T Z
50 ft – 15 m	P Z C K
40 ft – 12 m	S S J Z F
30 ft – 9 m	E Y J F X S
20 ft – 6 m	Q J H A L S E E
15 ft – 4.5 m	A Z R Y Y Y X Q P S

Made in the USA
Monee, IL
08 July 2022